THE BOOTCAMP BLUEPRINT

HOW PERSONAL TRAINERS CAN MAKE 6 FIGURES A YEAR, WORKING 60 MINS A DAY

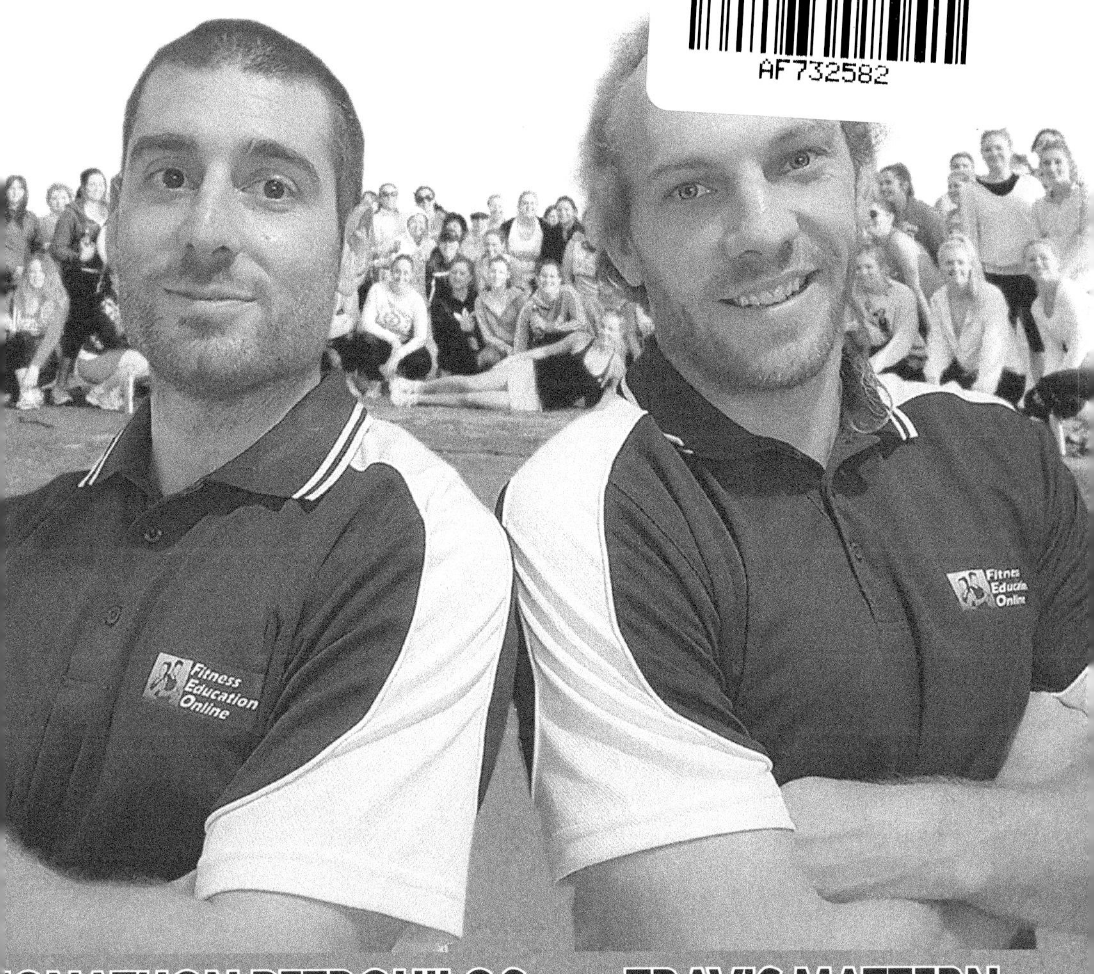

JONATHON PETROHILOS
TRAVIS MATTERN

First published by Busybird Publishing 2018

ISBN
Print: 978-1-925830-34-7
Ebook: 978-1-925830-36-1

Cover image: Busybird Publishing
Cover design: Busybird Publishing
Layout and typesetting: Busybird Publishing
Editor: Laura McCluskey

Busybird Publishing
2/118 Para Road
Montmorency, Victoria
Australia 3094
www.busybird.com.au

Testimonials

Adrian Hallam, PT:

'Your online VIP membership is the best community and best money I've ever spent. Jono and Travis are legends. I work alone, so your online community makes me feel like I'm not on my own. My membership is the best personal and professional investment I've ever made!'

Marckus Fenwick:

'I've been using the VIP program to set up my first 10-week bootcamp. Currently in Week 6. I've got 20 new members and about 12 to 16 per class. I do boxing Mondays, Thursdays, and bootcamp circuit, etc., Tuesday, Wednesday, Friday and Saturday mornings. It's great. I'm starting to repeat the classes with modified movements. The members haven't noticed. I'm getting great feedback. The content is great and Jono is on hand to answer any questions. As a long time fitness professional, I've found this as a great resource for my business. Highly recommend.'

Deborah Byrne:

'I've just completed the online essential social media course and can honestly say that its content far exceeded my expectations. The knowledge I've gained in such a short period of time has actually been more beneficial to my business than a $2500 mentoring course I completed last year. Although I haven't personally met Travis or Jono, I feel like they're both equally enthusiastic about the fitness industry. Their videos are packed full of information, are well presented and professional. It is blatantly obvious that they're both genuine and happy to share all of their expertise and knowledge in order for your business to be a success. Thank you guys, will definitely be signing up for more courses in the future.'

Ashy Evans:

'Ashy Bines here! I've known Jono from Fitness Education Online for a long time now, and we've worked pretty closely together in the past and he knows a thing or two about running a successful bootcamp! If you're a trainer looking to grow your bootcamp, I'd definitely recommend talking to Jono – easygoing, fun, and doesn't complicate things!'

Chantal Brodrick, host of The Fitness Business Podcast:

'I wanted to congratulate Jono and Travis on the fantastic community you are building for Fitness Education Online. The live videos in your community Facebook Group are excellent, the content is always so relevant and practical – it's clear you know the PT and bootcamp market inside out! Thank you for all the work you do to support fitness professionals in our industry.'

Jane O'Garey:

'Love your program!! For anyone thinking about doing the Level 1 and 2 in Bootcamp, DO IT!! Jono 'J-Z' Petrohilos knows what he is talking about, he has helped me get 54 ladies sign up to my first ever 10-week bootcamp at Rise and Shine Fitness Leeton. Now the ball is in my court and execution is key!!'

Jennelle Simpson:

'My name is Nell and I am a PT who specializes in training women over 40. I have been learning how to run an online bootcamp while running my normal group fitness and the information is wonderful. I spent 18k with another mob and their content and online was nowhere up to your level of practical doable information that has boosted my income and my sense of leadership. Would thoroughly recommend this course and the community.'

Sarah Jorgensen:

'I was struggling to get clients but after just one phone call everything became clear. I went back to the drawing board, wrote up my sales pitch, and practised, practised, practised. Went into the gym today and not only did I sign up a guy, but I sold him a 10-session package upfront. That alone gave me so much confidence that I went and nailed another client half an hour later. Couldn't have done it without your good advice and extremely helpful FB page. Thank you so much. Looking forward to building my business now!'

Jess Delmege:

'Only 2 weeks in and thanks to Fitness Education Online I've gone from 10 direct debit bootcamp clients to 26, and 6 new PT clients. I had been struggling for months before. Now with a brand new hyped up gym opening near me, I almost shut my business down. Well not anymore. Onwards and upwards to reach 50 new direct debit clients is my next goal. I can't wait to keep studying.'

Michelle Wright:

'I am Mish, the owner of Mishfit and the Business Development Manager at Curves Australia & NZ, and I present regularly at different fitness conferences on Women's health and business. Over the last couple of years, I have been working closely with Fitness Education Online and believe that they care deeply about providing great support and commitment to their community and care about providing education for Women's health – which is routinely overlooked. The folk at Fitness Education Online work with the highest of integrity and I think they do a great job!'

Sarah Skehan:

'My bootcampers are on their 8th week (final week) of this round. I followed Jono 'J-Z' Petrohilos bootcamp drills and now they want MORE! I had the girls pleading for me to continue 'til Christmas, sooo I just added another three weeks on! Thanks so much, Jono! You are a champ! And I should add that I'm getting new clients joining, too! Why re-invent the wheel when it works!'

Tracy Kingsbury:

'I messaged you about me doing an info session for my first bootcamp ever and you rang me with some advice. Well, 23 turned up for info session and 22 have paid in advance. One apologized stating she would love to do it, however she feels her body was not up to it. First session tomorrow morning, yay! Thank you! Thank you! Thank you!'

Trinity Roberts Brial:

'OMG, the Online Essentials Social Media Course is *amazing! I'm really enjoying it, and funnily enough, it feels more relevant and is so much more enjoyable* than the $8000 Diploma *I've almost finished with another company. Seriously, I highly recommend the* Online Essentials Social Media Course *to everyone!'*

Dedication

To the personal trainer who knows what it's like to start work at 5am every morning, finish work at 9pm every night, work weekends, not take holidays because you're scared your clients will leave, get underpaid and overworked – you've got two choices:

1. Get out of the industry and get a 'real job'.
2. Educate yourself so you can make fitness your full-time career, and live the lifestyle you want.

This book is dedicated to Number 2.

Contents

Jono's Story

'Failure is not the opposite to success,
it's part of success'
— Ariana Huffington

Before we get started, I want to share my story, and what I've been through in bootcamp. I have a reputation as being the 'go-to guy' when it comes to running a bootcamp, but it hasn't always been like that.

My background is actually in Exercise Physiology, and after completing my degree the goal was to work in a hospital with cardiac rehab patients. Obviously you need some experience working with the general public before a hospital is going to give you a job with the high-risk patients, so I started working at a gym on the floor. I thought it would be great – I'd have some fun, get some experience, train some people ... but I spent most of the time cleaning the treadmills, and doing the bathrooms checks.

One time, I had to trim the carpet hairs, because apparently it's a hazard when they're too long. I had to get down on my hands and knees and trim them with scissors! It's actually a pretty hard job, and really humiliating.

I spent a few years at this gym, and at the time I couldn't wait to get out of there! Looking back now, though, I wouldn't trade that experience for the world, because although it was hard work and minimum wage, I gained valuable experience.

A few years into my career an opportunity came up for me to manage a local bootcamp franchise. The *Seek* advertisement said 90% of the managers at this franchise make more than $75,000 a year working one hour a day (Monday to Saturday). I wasn't even making that $75,000 working 40 hours a week on the gym floor! So I took that opportunity head on, and was lucky enough to get the job!

Happy days, right? NO! When I first started running bootcamps I sucked at it, because here's the thing; no one really teaches you how to run a bootcamp. I had my degree in Exercise Physiology, a degree in Sports Science, my Cert III and IV in Fitness, I'd been working in gyms for five years, I'd taught group fitness classes, but when it came to running my own bootcamp, I had no idea what I was doing.

So I sucked ... and I mean *really* sucked! This is how bad I was – this franchise had 75 different locations across Australia and New Zealand, and each location was ranked 1-75 based on their retention, with 1st the best, and 75th the worst. Out of 75 different locations, take a guess at where I ranked. 35th? 45th? 17th?

I was ranked 75th!

I'm competitive; if I come second at something, I'm upset. If I come third at something, I'm very, very upset. If I come fourth at something, I'm borderline depressed. And I came 75th! I knew the trainer who was ranked at 74, and they sucked – but even they were smoking me! It wasn't good for my confidence. I was better at keeping the stats of how bad I was than actually running the bootcamp ... that says something.

To top it off, at the start of every year there was a national convention where all 75 franchise managers would attend. I didn't want to go; I was self-conscious as it is, because as a trainer, I'm not the biggest, the strongest, the fastest, or the sexiest (actually, maybe I was the sexiest – just kidding)!

Plus, I was the worst trainer there – in my mind, and statistically. I was hoping that I broke my leg, or got seriously injured so that I didn't have to go to this convention (not a joke, I would have literally preferred to have broken my leg than go). But I thought if I don't go, I'm going to get fired. If I do go, *maybe* I'll get fired, but maybe I'll keep my job and even learn a thing or two. Lucky for me I ended up going, because at this convention I met the head of the franchise who become my very first mentor and changed my life.

After hearing my mentor's story. I made a commitment to myself: for the next 12 months: I was going to do everything in my power to make sure that I ran the best bootcamp possible. I was going to do some courses in bootcamps, speak to successful trainers and see what they were doing, participate in their classes, hire a business coach, read books and watch YouTube videos on anything and everything that could help me on training, business, marketing, group dynamics confidence, personal development, etc. (and you will find a recommended reading list at the end of this book to get you started!)

It was a big change for me because none of my friends or family ran their own businesses, so their jobs were clock on/clock off! None of them would hire business coaches, or read Tony Robbins books, but I did! It was hard work, but I loved every minute of it!

Fast forward to 12 months later when I went to the next convention, and take a guess where I was ranked. 27th? 15th? 5th?

I was ranked 1st!

It was a big moment for me, and that journey from 75th to 1st in 12 months taught me a lot about myself and about bootcamp, but I wanted to keep going. Being #1 in the franchise was great, but now that I had a taste, I wanted to be the #1 bootcamp instructor in the world, so I dedicated my life to knowing anything and everything about running a successful bootcamp. Along the way other trainers started to approach me. They'd say, 'Jono, your bootcamp's always packed, you've got such a high retention rate – how do you do it?'

I spoke to my good friend (and now business partner at Fitness Education Online) Travis Mattern. At the time, Travis was a full-time teacher, and the Head Trainer at my bootcamp. He was (and still is) one of the only trainers I trusted to run bootcamp sessions for my clients.

I said, 'Travis, a lot of people are asking me questions about how to grow a bootcamp. I know you're a teacher and also an awesome bootcamp instructor. I'm thinking we should put a course together for personal trainers who want to run a successful bootcamp.' What do you think?'

Travis said, 'I go to a lot of these other courses for personal trainers, and they are ok, but I think we could do a better job! Let's do it!'

From there, we nutted it out and put together an online course for personal trainers who want to grow their bootcamp, consisting of everything we'd learned in our journey; the thousands of hours of teaching, studying, watching, and reading all put together in one course – and Fitness Educational Online was born. It all grew from there – we put out more and more courses, helped more and more trainers, and now we're one of the top education providers in the world for trainers who want to grow their bootcamp.

My goals have changed slightly, now. I'm no longer running a bootcamp on my own, because my goal is no longer to be the best bootcamp instructor in the world. Now I want to be the person who can help other trainers grow their bootcamps, and the person who runs the best courses for personal trainers. That's why Travis and I put this book together, and it's the perfect place for you to get started.

At the end of each chapter, you'll receive:

» Some Action Tasks.
» Some FAQ's.
» A comparison between two different bootcamps, labelled Bootcamp A and Bootcamp B. Bootcamp A is your 'average' bootcamp, the one that most trainers run and struggle to make a living from. Bootcamp B is the one that makes six-figures a year, working 60mins a day.
» Suggestions on where to go for more information on that chapter.

The Mindset of a Six-Figure Trainer

'Whether you think you can or whether you think you can't, you're right.'

— Henry Ford

If you don't have the right mindset, you can learn every trick in this book and you'll still fail. You can have the best workouts, all the best marketing, and thousands of followers on your social media, but if your mindset isn't right and you don't believe you can make six-figures a year working 60mins a day, guess what – you won't!

I could write a whole book on mindset, but there's thousands and thousands of books out there already. What I want to cover in this chapter is just three major points, and if you can master them, you'll run a six-figure bootcamp.

PRINCIPLE 1: The biggest difference between successful people and unsuccessful people is that successful people take 110% responsibility and accountability for everything in their life, whereas an unsuccessful person will blame someone or something else.

I believe this is the most important principle in life. I can tell straight away if a trainer is going to be successful based on this. Let me break down what I mean.

If something bad happens to a successful person, they're going to look at that situation and say, 'What did I do to cause that?' or, 'What can I learn from that?'

If something bad happens to an unsuccessful person, they're going to look for someone / something else to blame.

I learned this the hard way, because when I first started running a bootcamp, it was rubbish. I had low numbers, low retention, and I was struggling – but it wasn't *my* fault: there's too much competition in my area, there's a gym or bootcamp on every corner, it's winter, it's cold and rainy in Sydney, this franchise doesn't give me a lot of leads, and the leads they give me they never sign up anyway.

Can you see what was going on there? I was never going to be successful with that attitude, because I was doing the 'unsuccessful person' thing, not taking any responsibility and blaming everyone else but myself.

But as soon as I heard about this method (one of the first lessons my mentor taught me) I flicked the switch and started taking responsibility. From there, everything changed for me.

So, my mindset changed – it's NOT

- » the competition's fault that my bootcamp sucks, it's my fault that I haven't done enough to be better than the competition. As soon as I stopped blaming the competition and started taking ownership and responsibility for my own business, my numbers skyrocketed.
- » the franchise's fault that I'm not getting a lot of leads and that those leads aren't signing up. It's my fault because I don't do any of my own marketing. I should learn how to market myself.
- » the weather's fault that no one comes to training, it's my fault that I haven't done enough to not make the weather an issue. I solved that issue by renting out a school hall for $20 a session.

I've got a saying in my life now: 'There's no blaming, there's no complaining. If anything happens in my life, it's a direct result of something that I've done'. I'll look at the situation and say, 'Okay, what did I do to cause it, and what can I learn from this, so it never happens again?' This isn't just business, this is with everything in my life.

I was heading to a gym session with my personal trainer, Hanna, at 8am on a Tuesday morning. I was stuck in traffic, so I was going to text Hanna and say, 'I'm going to be 10 minutes late, because of traffic.' But then I thought, *I'm being a hypocrite if I say that*. It's not the traffic's fault, it's my fault.

My session is in peak-hour time, and I live in Sydney – of course there's going to be traffic. I should have left 10 minutes earlier, and even if I'd gotten there early, I could have used those extra minutes productively; answering emails, checking Facebook, replying to messages, etc.

PRINCIPLE 2: Successful people don't 'try' to do things.

I first heard about this exercise from Jack Canfield from *The Secret*. It goes like this:

Jack tells everyone to put their pen down in front of them. He then asks everyone to pick up their pen, so they do. At this point the audience is thinking, 'Okay, that was easy.' He then asks everyone to put their pen down in front of them again. This time Jack says, 'Don't pick it up, just TRY and pick it up. Ready? 1, 2, 3, go. Everyone TRY and pick up your pen.'

The audience is all confused; a couple of people picked up their pen, a couple of people didn't pick it up, but most people are saying, 'Jack, what are you talking about? You're not making sense. If you want us to pick it up, just say so and we'll pick it up. If you don't want us to pick it up, that's cool. You can't TRY to pick up a pen.

And his response is, 'You're spot on, but unfortunately, that's how a lot of people live their lives. Instead of doing something, they TRY to do it – and it makes no sense.

I thought about it, and realised it happens a lot in my life. A lot of people say, 'Jono, I really want to lose weight, so I'm going to TRY to go to the gym every day this week.'

How can you TRY and go to the gym? What do you do? Do you get up off the couch and then realize you're stuck to it and can't move? Or do you get in the car to drive to the gym, but then somehow you magically end up at KFC? It doesn't make sense. If you want to lose weight, don't TRY and go to the gym every day this week – actually GO to the gym every day this week!

Now that I speak to a lot of other personal trainers, a lot of them say things like, 'I really want to grow my business, so I'm going to try and read for an hour every day.' How can you TRY to read? Either you read, or you don't. What do you do? You open up a book and then the wind just keeps blowing the pages closed so you can't read it? Or do you open the book to read it, and you find out it's in another language? It doesn't make sense. If you want to grow your business, don't TRY and read for an hour every day – actually read for an hour every day!

What we're really saying with the word 'try' is that we only half want something.

I always ask my bootcampers on Fridays if they'll be coming to the following morning's 7am session, and a lot my participants say, 'Oh yeah, Jono, I'm gonna TRY and make it.' Whenever they say that, I know they're not coming, and they even know they're not coming. They just feel bad telling me they're not coming, so they use the word 'try' because it gives them a bit of an out. It's like, 'Well, I didn't 100% commit to Jono, so he can't kick up a stink if I didn't come, but I'm not going to say no to his face because I feel like an idiot and he might get upset.'

What you're really saying is, 'Hey, I'd prefer to stay in bed than go and reach my goals' or, 'I'd prefer to go out drinking tonight than wake up early tomorrow.' No one wants to say those things aloud, or even admit to thinking like that!

PRINCIPLE 3: Successful people see failure as a positive.

A major thing that stops people from being successful is they're scared of failing. We grow up thinking failing is a bad thing; in school you're taught that if you get something right, that's good, and if you get something wrong, that's bad. I think that's complete opposite. There's no shame in getting something wrong; it's the best way to learn! And this is a big difference between successful people and unsuccessful people.

The unsuccessful person won't take a risk because they are scared to fail; the successful person will take the risk because they know the risk will either pay off, or they'll learn something. The only reason I'm this position now is because I've failed more than anyone else I know – this might sound funny, but I love failing! Having said that, I've actually removed the word 'failure' from my vocabulary and replaced it with 'learning experience' – that way I never fail, I either win, or I learn; both of which are positive things.

So, if you want to do something, do it. Don't let the fear hold you back, because only one of two things can happen: either you do it and you're successful, or you do it and you fail, but you learn something and you're better off for it. The more you fail, the more you learn. My biggest regret is that I didn't fail more when I was younger!

FAQ

'Jono/Travis, I believe all this stuff and it makes sense, but I'm just not sure if I can do it. Is it really possible?'

Our answer to this is simple. You can either have results, or you can have excuses. You can't have both, so choose wisely. If you want to have excuses, that's fine, keep them coming, but hey you're not going to be successful. If you want to get the results and be successful and awesome, scrap that excuse and find a way.

If you don't believe it's possible, you'll never be able to do it. But if you believe it's possible, you'll find a way!

Action Tasks

1. Take 110% responsibility for EVERYTHING in your life.
2. Remove the word 'try' from your vocabulary.
3. Remove the word 'failure' from your vocabulary, and replace it with 'learning experience'.

Bootcamp A vs Bootcamp B

Instructor A's business is not growing as quick as they'd like. It's not their fault though: it's winter so the numbers are low, Facebook changed their algorithm so no one is seeing their posts, and the people that are inquiring aren't answering their phone. They are still trying to do things to grow their bootcamp: posting on social media once a week, they are trying to read books on marketing and sales, and they are trying to network with local people in the area.

Instructor B's business is not growing as quick as they like. They understand it's their own fault; they didn't do enough marketing in summer to prepare for the lower amount of inquiries in winter, they didn't learn enough about social media to know about the Facebook algorithm changes. They, however, are still going to grow their bootcamp; they are posting on social media every week, they are reading about sales and marketing every day, and they are networking every day with local people in their area.

Books to read

- *Think and Grow Rich* by Napolean Hill
- *Awaken The Giant Within* by Tony Robbins
- *The Success Principles* by Jack Canfield
- *The Secret* by Rhonda Byrne
- *You Were Born Rich* by Bob Proctor

Why Bootcamp is Your Best Option!

In this chapter I'm going to explain why bootcamps are your best option *if done correctly*! I teach a very specific method of running a bootcamp, which is: 'Make Six Figures a Year Working 60Mins a Day'.

There's two key components to this model:

1. Making six figures a year (approx. $2000 per week).
4. Working 60mins a day.

Whenever I tell that to people they're like, 'Haha, yeah I wish, but you can't do that. That's a dream.'

And I'm like, 'Well, actually no, it's not that hard if you structure everything properly.'

All you need to do is run one bootcamp session a day (Monday to Saturday) and charge $50 per week (approx. $10 per session, which is very reasonable). Then all you need is 40 clients in there, and you're making $2000 a week. If you feel like 40 clients is too big of a goal to start with, that's fine – just use 20 clients, and you'll still make $1000 a week working 60mins a day.

So, why bootcamp? Why choose this activity, when there's so many different things we can do as personal trainers?

We can do

- » bootcamps.
- » one-on-one personal training.
- » small group / semi-private training.
- » online personal training.
- » sell supplements / pyramid schemes.
- » and, of course, underwear modelling.

To see why I recommend bootcamp, let's compare it with **one-on-one personal training**.

At the time of writing this book, an average one-on-one PT session is approx. $50 for a 45min session, so if a personal trainer wants to make $1000 week, they will need 20 clients (or 20 sessions). Let's average it out, and say each session is actually an hour. The personal trainer needs to work 20 hours to make $1000 a week.

If a bootcamp instructor wants to make $1000 a week, they will also need 20 clients, but they are only working 5-6 hours a week!

Which one sounds like a better deal? Make $1000 in 5-6 hours a week, or make $1000 in 20 hours a week?

Let's say $1000 isn't enough – we want to make six figures a year, so we've got to make $2000 a week. The bootcamp instructor needs another 20 clients (40 total). That's fine, they get another 20 clients and they still only need to work 5-6 hours a day, whereas the PT now has to work 40 hours a week.

40 hours of PT? That's a full-time job, and is almost impossible. Office workers complain that 40 hours is too hard, and they sit in an office. Imagine training someone for 40 hours a week. Also, that's with no benefits; not only are you training people for 40 hours a week, there's no super, there's no holidays, there's no retirement funds, there's no sick leave, there's no annual leave … it's just pure work!

Now, what if you want to go next level, and your goal is to make $5000 a week (100 clients)

If you're running a bootcamp, cool, you need to get those 100 clients down there – but you're still only working 5-6 hours a week. If you're a PT and you want to have 100 clients, you've got to work 100 hours a week. My maths is rubbish, but is there even 100 hours in a week?

You might be reading this and thinking, '100 clients? Jono, I can't run a bootcamp with 100 clients! I'll need to hire 4-5 trainers to do that, and that's going to cause all sorts of headaches!'

Well … not really. Let me simplify it!

If you've got 100 clients registered for your bootcamp, not every client is coming to every session. Most people train three times a week, or thereabouts, so if you're running six sessions a week, you're probably going to get half the numbers there. Therefore, for those six sessions a week, out of the 100 clients you're probably going to get 50 people per session.

In my opinion, even 50 clients to one trainer is too much. I don't like to train more than 20-25 people at once, so if I had 50 people per session, I would hire another trainer to run the session with me and then split the group up in two, so each trainer is in charge of 25 people. That's achievable, right? You'd pay that trainer a flat fee of $50 per session, so if you've got 100 clients paying $50 per week, you'll earn $5000 and your other trainer will take $300 ($50 x 6) – you profit $4700. Not bad!

The one hour a day part of my system is important, and this is the mistake a lot of trainers make. They run multiple sessions a day, e.g. one at 6am, another at 9:30am, and then another session at 6:30pm. The major reason this doesn't work is if you're running multiple sessions a day, you don't have the time to run a six-figure bootcamp!

To run a 6 figure bootcamp, it's not just about the session. Along with providing an amazing session you need to

- work on your sales and marketing (so you can get 40 people registered).
- work on your support OUTSIDE of training (so you can KEEP the current clients you've got).
- further educate yourself by doing courses and reading to stay on top of the game (otherwise you'll get stale).

Looking at a day with the '60mins a day' system, let's say you run your session at 6am Mon-Sat. By the time you finish your session, talk to clients, pack your car, and get home, it might be 7:30-8am. But at that point, you're done with work for the day! So you might spend a couple hours on your sales and marketing, a couple hours on your support, and then a couple hours on your education.

If you're running multiple sessions a day, you can't spend the same amount of time as the '60min a day' trainer on sales/marketing, support, and education because you're working all day!

It's a vicious cycle, because that trainer usually wants to grow their bootcamp and they know what they have to do to grow it, but 'they don't have time'.

So, the answer is: use the 60min a day model!

FAQ

'What about people who can't make that one timeslot? What happens for the people who can't make 6am sessions?'

There's two different ways you can run our system.

Option 1: The One Timeslot

You can pick one timeslot and run it at the same time every day, either 6am, 9:30am, or 6:30pm, depending on who you're targeting. If you want to target the before-work people, you'd want to train early morning every day – Monday to Friday at 6am, and Saturday at 7am.

If you want to target mums, train after school drop-off times – Monday to Friday at 9:30am, and Saturday at 7am.

If you want to target the after-work people, train after work finishes – Monday to Friday at 6:30pm, and Saturday at 7am.

With this system, some people are going to miss out, but that's ok. You just want to pick whichever timeslot you believe will be the most popular, and then spend all your efforts getting as many people down to it as possible!

Will you miss out on some clients because of it? Of course! But what often happens to trainers who run multiple sessions per day is something like this:

6am session – 10 participants

9:30am session – 3 participants

6:30pm session – 5 participants

That trainer would be better off scrapping the 9:30am and 6:30pm sessions. They'll lose some clients, but they gain their time back and they can spend that time on their business getting more people down to the 6am session!

Option 2: The Split Timeslot

Split your session timetable across different days. For example:

Monday/Wednesday/Friday – 6am

Tuesday/Thursday – 6:30pm

Saturday – 7am

Here you're hedging your bets. You're assuming most people only want to train three times a week and that they are either going to do M, W, F or T, T, S.

The advantage to this system is there is more variety; you can catch the morning people and the evening people.

This is usually the easier option when starting off. Both options can work, it just depends which way you want to go.

'Jono, Travis, you're saying you charge $50 per week for 5-6 sessions, but what happens if people can only make 1-2 sessions? How much do you charge for a casual, and how much do you charge for a 10-pack?

We don't do either. We don't do casuals, we don't do 10-packs. We run it as a 12-week challenge, $50 a week for the 12 weeks. It doesn't matter whether you attend one, or whether you attend five – it is what it is.

It's very strategic as well, because allowing casuals just doesn't work. We're all about value – we put a lot of time outside of the session to our clients (to ensure that they come back), and it's only worth our while to put in that time if we're getting paid at least $50 per week from each person. We could get a casual in for $15-$20 and not give them the support outside of the session, but we'd just feel bad doing that. To keep it simple, everyone pays $50 and gets an amazing service!

The other way we look at it is we're not charging per session; if you get into charging per session you're gone. It's $50 a week to be part of my community – you can come to as many sessions as you want, and you get all these extras, as well (we'll be discussing these later in the book).

Action Tasks

1. Choose the date you're going to kick off your 12-week challenge, and which timeslots your sessions are going to be (Option 1 or Option 2).
2. If you're already running a bootcamp with multiple sessions a day, see what you can cut out. Are there sessions where only 2-3 people are coming to every session? It might be best off just canning that session. Even if you lose a client or two, you've now got an hour or two to work on your sales and marketing, and pack up some of your more sessions.

3. If you're doing casuals or 10-packs, start to phase that out. If people are already paying those existing rates, then let that continue for a while, but any new person who signs up must do the $50 per week.

Bootcamp A vs Bootcamp B

Instructor A has 20 clients registered and runs three sessions a day. They want to grow their bootcamp, but are finding it hard because they keep running out of time to do the sales and marketing because they are spending all their time running their sessions and supporting their current clients. Instructor A also feels their sessions are getting a little stale because they don't have time to research new ideas.

Instructor B has 20 clients registered and runs one session a day. They finish work at 7am every morning, and spend a couple of hours working on supporting their current clients. They've still got plenty of time up their sleeve to work on sales and marketing, and continue to educate themselves on new session ideas.

More information

We cover this in our Bootcamp CEC courses – to check them out, simply go to our website (www.fitnesseducationonline.com.au). Join our community Facebook Group (www.facebook.com/groups/fitnesseducationonline) where we have over 8000 trainers from all over the world discussing these topics.

How to Create a Bootcamp That Sells

'When you do more than you're paid to do, you will eventually be paid more for what you do.'

—Zig Ziglar

We're not talking about the actual workouts here (we'll get to that later). Most trainers are pretty good with their workouts – it's the things *outside* of the bootcamp sessions that let them down!

Let's compare two bootcamps to show you what I mean.

Bootcamp A:

» 12-Week Challenge (5-6 sessions a week).

» $50 a week.

Bootcamp B:

- 12-Week Challenge (5-6 sessions a week).
- $50 a week.
- Jono's 12-Week Home Program.
- Jono's Basic Nutrition Guidelines.
- Jono's Clean Eating Recipe eBook.
- Jono's Clean Eating Smoothie and Shake eBook.
- Jono's 7-Day Ab Program.
- Jono's 7-Day Booty Program.
- Access to Jono's VIP Facebook group.
- Cool extra challenges such as: Week 2 = No sugar challenge, Week 4 = Walking challenge, Week 6 = Bring a friend and invite them to take on the final six weeks, Week 8 = Fun-Run or obstacle course, Week 10 = Recipe sharing challenge, Week 12 = End of challenge celebration.

Which bootcamp do you think will be more popular?

Which bootcamp will be easier to sell? It's a no-brainer right?

Don't get intimidated by this. When I tell trainers this model, they often freak out and say they can't do it because it's too much, or they don't have time … all the usual excuses!

Let me break it down and simplify it into three main secrets:

- Electronic Programs
- Online Challenges
- Excursions

SECRET 1: ELECTRONIC PROGRAMS

The first aspect is the Electronic Programs (my Home Program, Basic Nutrition Guidelines, Clean Eating Recipe eBook, Clean Eating Smoothie and Shake eBook, 7-Day Ab Program, 7-Day Booty Program).

These are awesome because you only have to write them up once! You never have to do it again, but you can give it to every new client!

It's a great feeling to know you've done the work once, but continue getting paid for it again and again!

FAQ:

'Jono/Travis, what happens if someone signs up again for another 12-Week Challenge – don't you have to give them a new Home Program?'

No! The Home Program is for new clients, and it's more a sales tool to get people in the door!

Once they are in, it's up to me to use my magic and give them the best experience possible so that they sign up again!

That's what they come back for – the experience, not the free eBook!

'How do you have the time to put all that together?'

This is why we recommend only working one hour a day – so you have the time to do this!

We just slowly built all this up, starting with the 12-Week Home Program.

We hung back after training on Monday mornings every week and took a 5-10min video explaining what that week's 'home workout' would be for anyone who couldn't make the session. We did that every week for 12 weeks, and at the end we had our 12-Week Home Program!

'How do I put an eBook together?

We use www.fiverr.com, a website where you can hire freelancers to do pretty much anything you want done for a fee of $5! The first eBook we put together was my Clean Eating Recipe eBook.

We did a recipe challenge in the Facebook Group asking all my clients to share a recipe, and ended up with about 30 recipes. We sent them all to a person on fiverr, paid them $5, and they turned it into an eBook!

SECRET 2: ONLINE CHALLENGES

The Electronic Programs are good, but as they just provide clients with more info, I find the Online Challenges better because they are interactive and actually provide support, accountability, communication, and motivation outside of the session.

A lot of trainers are really good at providing those during in the session, but if you're running a bootcamp you've only got those people for one hour a day, if that.

If you can get your online community happening, it's going to do wonders for your bootcamp, and your retention.

Using the No-Sugar Challenge as an example, I'm going to break down how this hits all those points.

Jono 'j-z' Petrohilos is with Cindy Wunderlich and 14 others.
Admin · August 7, 2016 · Kogarah

14 Day No Sugar Challenge!

Starting tomorrow (Mon 8th August)!

Rules are simple

1: Tag your name in the comments section below
2: At the end of every day post the amount of sugar you had in that day in the "reply" section under your name (i'll do an example for myself so you know what i mean)

There's no "right" or "wrong" for the exact amount of sugar... Most natural foods have a couple grams in there so it's pretty much impossible to get "zero"... So the goal is just to get as low as possible!

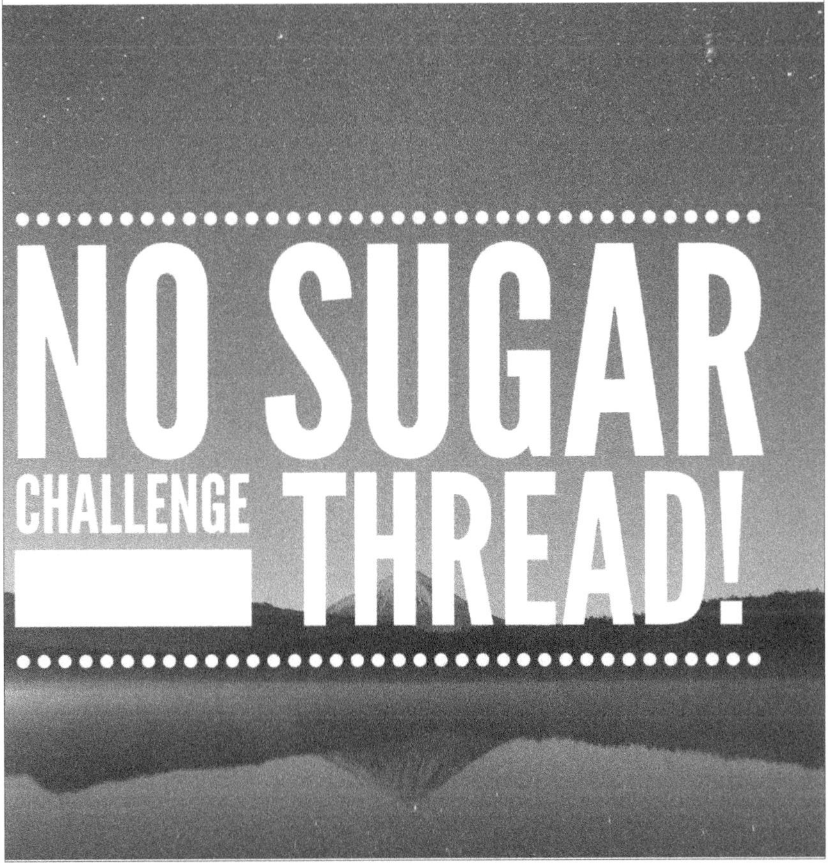

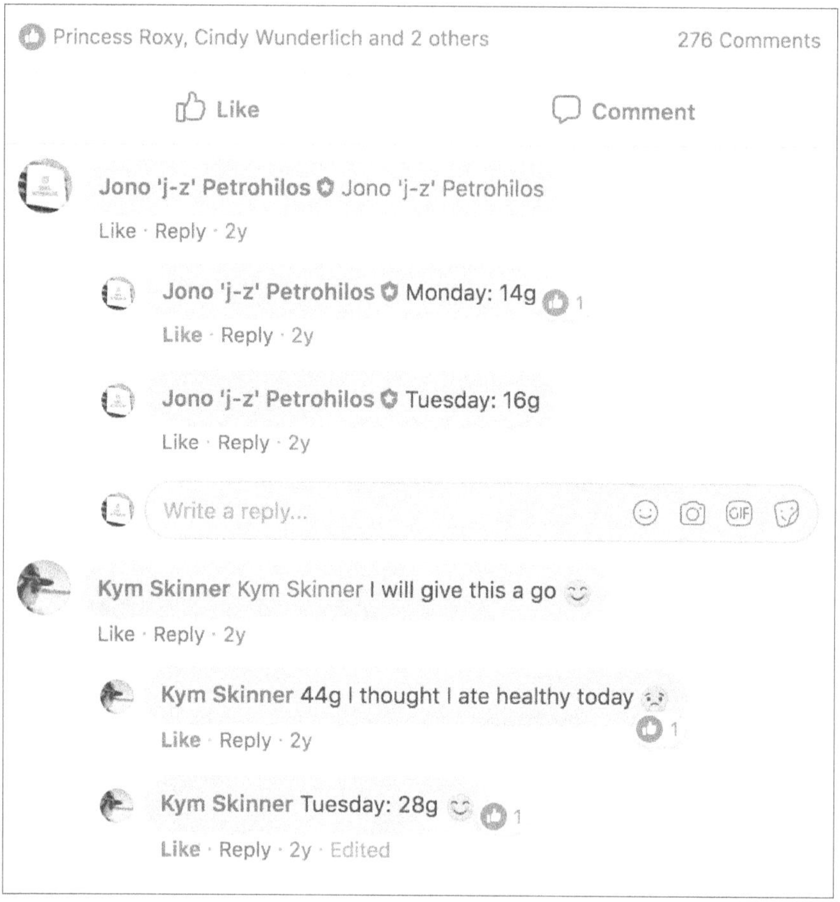

As you can see from these two images, it's pretty easy.

- Make a post in your Facebook Group saying, 'This week we're doing the No-Sugar Challenge. The goal is to have as little sugar as possible for the whole week. Comment your name, and the amount of grams of sugar you have each day.'
- Check the thread each day.
- Respond to each participant's comment with encouragement, 'Good work'.
- If someone forgets a day, tag them in the post to remind them. Say, 'Hey, Maria – you said you were going to do this challenge, but you haven't tracked anything. What's going on?'

In this post, we have a few things at play.

Motivation: People are going to be more motivated to do it because everyone is participating. Not many people would do it just for the fun, but if it's part of the bootcamp activities they'll be more interested in taking part.

Community: As I said above, people will be more likely to do it as it's a group challenge. The challenge is also a bonding experience to bring them together as a group, especially if they invite their friends and family to participate.

Accountability: Studies show that just by tracking your food, you're going to be more careful of what you eat. This challenge means your clients are going to be more accountable to themselves. Tagging them if they forget to post adds another layer of accountability.

Support: Alone, people usually give up tracking their food after 1-2 days because it's boring. If there's someone (e.g. their trainer) supporting them, they are more likely to stay on track because they know someone else actually cares.

SECRET 3: EXCURSIONS

I do an excursion every month; so if it's a 12-Week Challenge, I plan three excursions for Week 4, Week 8, and Week 12 (can vary).

There's a party at the end of Week 12, and I could do a whole chapter on how to make that work. Put simply – really have a party! Have a dinner, maybe some drinks, play some games, give out some awards, make it fun, and give everyone a chance to bond outside of the training sessions! Don't underestimate this as a retention tool! I've had clients that were 50/50 about coming back to the next bootcamp, but just by going to that party and getting closer to the group, they decided to stay on.

You need to put effort into these excursions. Promote them so people will come, and actively do things to make it fun so that people aren't bored! Excursion options are endless; you can do Fun-Runs, obstacle courses, pole dancing, rock climbing, beach sessions, stair sessions, breakfasts, stand-up paddleboarding, trampolining, martial arts, canoeing, Sky Zone, to name a few!

It's also important that these excursions require you do it as 'teams' or 'partners'; things that people wouldn't/couldn't do on their own, outside of bootcamp. The obstacle courses are a perfect example of this. Not many people are going to do one of those on their own (unless they are already a trainer/fitness fanatic), but if they've got a group of friends doing it, they may give it a go!

There's a sense of accomplishment after doing activities like these – clients say, 'Wow, this bootcamp is awesome, it's giving me opportunities to do all these amazing things I've always wanted to do … so I better keep going with it!'

The seasons are going to matter as well, because obviously water activities work better in the summer. You can use that to your advantage; summer challenges can be the beach and water challenges or excursions, and winter can be for the more indoor ones.

I can't stress how important these things are – especially the Online Challenges and the excursions! I've had people in my bootcamp stay (and keep paying), even though they haven't come to a session in weeks, because they come to the Fun-Run, the breakfasts, they're in the Facebook Group, they do the No-Sugar Challenge … they're happy to pay even though they're not coming to the sessions because they're getting so much value from everything else!

FAQ

'I'm not qualified in nutrition. How do I stay within my scope of practice?'

The current scope of practice for a personal trainer requires them to be 'able to provide basic nutrition guidance, consistent with the national guidelines.' (Fitness Australia).

Look at what we give out:

- » BASIC nutrition guidelines that we get straight from the guidelines of Healthy Eating! That way we know we're within scope.
- » Clean Eating Recipes/Smoothies/Shakes are just recipes/ideas. It's not a specific meal plan saying this is what my clients have to have! It's just saying, 'If you're ever out of ideas, here's a few!'
- » The challenges (e.g. no sugar, hydration, etc.) is more about support, motivation, accountability. We're not saying, 'You need to have less than [this] amount of sugar' or anything like that.

'Do I have to do this again every 12 weeks?'

Not really ...

With the Electronic Programs, you do them once, then that's it – never again.

Yes, our participants do the same challenges every 12 weeks, but to be honest, they love it! You'll only do each challenge four times a year, so by the time it comes around, you're looking forward to it!

It's similar with the excursions; we know what excursions work and which ones don't, so we do use similar ones. But we don't do EXACTLY the same excursions every challenge for two main reasons:

» The season: In summer/spring my excursions are more water/outdoor-based (e.g. SUP, beach sessions, canoeing, etc.). In winter/autumn my excursions are more indoor-based (e.g. trampolining, pole dancing, martial arts.)
» Timing of Fun-Runs/obstacle courses: These are usually on certain dates every year, so we plan around that.

Action Tasks

1. Plug in what excursions you're going to do, and when.
2. Plug in what online challenges you're going to do, and when.
3. Slowly start putting together your online programs.

Bootcamp A vs Bootcamp B

Instructor A's bootcamp is $50 a week for 6 sessions. They are struggling to get new clients, even though they are a really good trainer.

Instructor B's bootcamp is $50 a week for 6 sessions PLUS a heap of electronic programs, excursions, and online challenges. They are finding it easy to get new clients.

More information

This is the sort of content we cover in our Bootcamp and Social Media CEC courses – to check them out, simply go to our website (www.fitnesseducationon line.com.au).

Also make sure you join our community Facebook Group (www.facebook.com/groups/fitnesseducationonline) where we have over 8000 trainers from all over the world discussing these topics.

How to Get As Many Clients As You Want!

You can be the best bootcamp instructor in the world, but if you don't know how to sell and market yourself, you're going to be sitting alone in that park doing push-ups.

I've said it's not that hard to get a six-figure bootcamp. All you need is 40 clients paying you $50 a week, over 12 weeks – and there's your $2000 a week.

By now you're probably asking, 'Jono, where am I going to find 40 people to fill that bootcamp up?'

Well, it's actually a lot easier than what you think. There's no surprises here. The easiest way to pack out your bootcamp is via a good social media strategy. Yes, there's other things you can do as well that compliment that, but this is the easiest, fastest, and the most effective way.

It's a gold mine – we've never had this opportunity before, where people are bumping into poles on the street because they're so busy on their phone. We don't know how long it's going to be around, so let's make the most of it.

The biggest advantages of social media are that it's instant, affordable, and it's scalable. You can make a Facebook post right now for free, and people can start inquiring! It's not like back in the day when you had to put an ad in the phonebook.

Not only would you have to pay thousands of dollars, it wouldn't come out until the next year when the new copy came out, and it wasn't even targeted! Now with social media you can target the exact people you want, and if you want to grow quicker you can put some dollars behind it, not thousands, to promote your message. It's just so powerful, and it's so important that we learn it.

There's two parts to my strategy: social media strategy, and the bootcamp strategy, and they work hand-in-hand.

My social media strategy breaks into three parts:

» Step 1: 'Facebook Ads' to generate leads (name, number, email).
» Step 2: 'Phone calls' to see if the lead is interested in joining.
» Step 3: 'Email Marketing and Community Facebook Group' to nurture the prospects who didn't join from the phone call.

Let's delve into these in a little more detail.

Step 1: Facebook Ads

The easiest way to get leads from Facebook is via a 'Facebook Lead Ad'. This is an ad that appears on your News Feed where when you click 'learn more'. You then enter in your details to get more info. This is by far the most effective strategy on Facebook for two main reasons:

1. You now have the person's phone number.
You can give them a call and have a chat person to person! This is so powerful because people are FLOODED with fitness posts on Facebook; every second person is trying to sell them some weight-loss product, so they ignore most of them. If you can actually have a genuine conversation with them – you've got a chance. Calling off a Facebook ad is about the easiest way you can sell, because you've specifically targeted this person, you know they've seen your ad and opted to learn more, and they've entered in their contact details! That's about as hot of a lead as you can get.

2. You've got this persons details for life!
Even if they don't sign up for this challenge, when your next challenge comes around you can give them another call, or just send out a bulk text, or an email! All for free! But, if you didn't have their contact details you'd have to keep paying Facebook for ads.

Let me give you an example:

You've got a 12-Week Challenge coming up, so you put $500 on a Facebook Ad campaign. You get 50 leads (name, number, email), but only one signs up. You could look at that and think that was a waste of money, but I look at that differently. I say, 'Awesome, I made my money back because now I have 50 leads, and sooner or later those 50 leads are going to sign up with me – providing I nurture them properly!'

If you do that every 12 weeks, 12 months later you've now got 200 people on your database. You're basically building your list for free!

STEP 2: Sales calls

'Sales' can be a scary word for a lot of trainers because they think they need to be sleazy/pushy, but it is the exact opposite – sales is about helping people!

I want to stress that if you want to grow your bootcamp, then phone sales is the most important part! A lot of people get caught up in social media and lead generation, which is important, but if those followers/leads aren't paying you then it means absolute nothing!

I recommend hiring a sales coach to help with your selling. A good sales coach will not cost you money, it will make you money!

STEP 3: Email Marketing and Community Facebook Group

Two examples:

1: Bootcamp A gets 50 leads, but 49 don't register. 12 weeks later, Instructor A sends out a bulk email asking those 49 to join for the next 12-Week Challenge.

That may work.

2: Bootcamp B gets 50 leads, but 49 don't register. Every week for 12 weeks, Instructor B sends out an email giving the lead a health/fitness tip for free. Instructor B also adds the lead to their 'community Facebook Group' where they post a video every week giving a free health/fitness tip. 12 weeks later, Instructor B sends out a bulk email asking those 49 to join for the next 12-Week Challenge.

Bootcamp B will get a much better response because they've been building a rapport for 12 weeks.

In terms of the email and community Facebook group, they're whole other beasts on their own, the best thing to do would be to watch what I do – join my email list and my community Facebook group and see how I manage both.

That's the 3-Step system, and it's important that you put it in place with your bootcamp strategy, as well. This is why the 12-Week Challenge works so well, because the hardest part of running a bootcamp, or being a personal trainer, is sales and marketing whilst also serving your clients at the same time.

2-3 weeks before a challenge begins, grind hard on your sales and marketing, put a few dollars in your Facebook ads, send out some emails, make some Facebook posts, and make a heap of sales calls. Then for the next 12 weeks, you just make sure you give these people an amazing service so that every single one of them signs back up again.

Then you do the same thing at around Week 10 – slow down on the support a bit because by that time people have already decided if they will come back or not, grind hard on your sales and marketing, get a whole heap of new people in, and then give those people an amazing service. We'll cover this a bit more on the retention side of things.

The other advantage of a 12-Week Challenge is that there's a set start point; when you call someone, they can't say, 'Oh yeah, I'll think about it.' If it starts next week you can simply say, 'Are you in, or are you out?'

FAQ

This is starting to get confusing. Where do I start?

Just pick one thing at a time, and master that before moving onto something else. That's what we did. First we learned about Facebook Ads, then Facebook Groups, then email marketing, then phone sales.

You can learn it yourself via YouTube / books. We recommend doing a course in each topic to learn. You'll spend a lot of time and money fiddling around if you try yourself, whereas if you do a course, you'll spend a few dollars on the course, but you'll save money and time long-term.

Bootcamp A vs Bootcamp B

Instructor A is not getting any new clients, they are posting on social media, and even occasionally boosting their posts, but no one is signing up.

Instructor B is constantly getting new clients, they have a Facebook Lead ad running, and people are constantly inquiring. Instructor B calls all these inquiries, some register, but most don't. The ones who don't register get added to the email list and the community Facebook Group, and receive emails / posts regularly.

Action Tasks

1. Learn how to use Facebook Ads.
2. Learn how to sell over the phone.
3. Learn how to use Email Marketing.
4. Learn how to use Facebook Groups.

More information

This is the sort of content we cover in our Bootcamp and Social Media CEC courses – to check them out, simply go to our website (www.fitnesseducationon line.com.au). Also make sure you join our community Facebook Group (www.facebook.com/groups/fitnesseducationonline) where we have over 8000 trainers from all over the world discussing these topics.

Books to read

Secrets to Closing the Sale by Zig Ziglar

Sell or Be Sold by Grant Cardone

Psychology of Selling by Brian Tracey

The Psychology of Influence and Persuasion by Robert Cialdini

The Greatest Salesmen in the World by OG Mandino

No BS Direct Marketing by Dan Kennedy

It's Not Who You Know, It's Who Knows You

'Originally the secret to success was "what you know". Then it was "who you know". Now, it's "who knows you".'

—David Averin

I love networking, probably because I'm pretty good at it. It's helped me over the years to become a very successful bootcamp instructor, a very successful entrepreneur, and a very successful business owner. I'm going to explain what networking is, how to do it, and the benefits of it.

There's an element of luck involved in success. Now, I'm not a huge fan of the word 'luck', but if you do the right things you can swing that luck in your favour. We've all seen people use luck to get to their position because they 'knew the right person'. Well, there's two ways you can react to that. You can either sit back and think, 'They only got successful because they knew the right person,' or go out and meet more people so that sooner or later you're going to meet the 'right person'.

I'm going to give you three strategies to help with this:

» Strategy 1: Meet as MANY people as possible!
» Strategy 2: Meet the RIGHT people!
» Strategy 3: ASSOCIATE with the right people!

Strategy 1: Meet as MANY people as possible

Instructor A is running a bootcamp and only knows 10 people in the local area.

Instructor B is running a bootcamp and knows 100 people in the local area.

Let's say it's a 20% hit ratio of people you know training with you.

Instructor A sends out 10 text messages to their friends in the area, and 20% want to join the bootcamp. Great, that's two clients.

Instructor B sends out 100 text messages to their friends in the area, and 20% want to join the bootcamp. That's 20 clients.

From a purely math side of things, it's a bigger advantage to know more people in your local area!

In the beginning I didn't go out and 'meet as many people as possible' to grow my business, I just did it for fun and as a result my business grew. Let me explain what I mean:

For about 2-3 years I worked full-time in a local gym on the gym floor. I did a bit of personal training and group fitness stuff, but most of my job was just on the floor. It's not always the most fun job; you're cleaning the treadmills, stacking the soda machine, and doing the bathroom checks. I thought, *If I've got to be here for 40 hours a week; how can I make this time fly?* Become good friends with every single person who comes in: members, staff, co-workers, managers, everyone! This gym was quite a big leisure center with pools, saunas, two receptions desks, basketball courts, kids programs, etc., so there were heaps of members and staff: receptionists, sales staff, personal trainers, group fitness instructions, gym floor, life guards, learn-to staff, café staff, etc.

I also thought about how good it would be for these gym members (and staff) to come to the gym/work and see someone who's one of their good friends? They're going to be more likely to enjoy the experience! On a purely selfish note for me, if I ever wanted to get a promotion, it would help if all the members and staff liked me. So, every person who I got on well with, I added to Facebook! This is so important for a few different reasons:

» This will deepen our 'bond'. Not only are we just 'gym friends' but we also connect outside of the gym (even if it's just online).
» We are now friends for 'life' (or until they block me)! Even if they change gyms, they'll still have a way to contact me.
» I can 'softly' promote my services. I don't want to promote my services to members of a gym while I'm working at that gym – I don't think it's ethical. But if I've got these people on Facebook and they happen to see my posts and contact me outside of the gym, I'm not going to turn them down.

When I started my first bootcamp I didn't want to tell the members what I was doing because it's not fair on the gym, but I told my colleagues at the leisure center and three of the receptionists signed up! Once my bootcamp started to pick up I cut down my hours at the gym, and then pretty much left completely.

Now that I was only working 60mins a day I had some more time up my hands. A new gym opened up down the road from me and was looking for group instructors. I had the time, so I signed up. Then I used exactly the same strategy; I taught group fitness classes, made sure I got on really well with all the members and staff, added anyone I got on with to Facebook, and just repeated the exact system. This has also become a personal thing; my 'life goal' is to become really good friends with every single person I meet, and then add them on Facebook. Everywhere I go, I'm armed with my phone. If you speak to me and we get along – I'm adding you to Facebook. The amount of friends/connections/ networks I've made from this strategy is the reason I'm in my current position.

In saying that, working in a gym isn't your only option. Maybe you don't want to do that, or maybe you want to do that PLUS more! The other popular one is school groups. I speak to a lot of trainers who want to start a bootcamp and know all the 'school mums'. Use the same strategy; get active in the school community, and meet the parents!

I don't have kids so I can't give advice there, but some other things I've done in the area was learn Spanish for a semester, salsa dancing for a semester, singing lessons for a term, and Toastmasters for a term. I don't go to these things to specifically grow my business, I go to learn some things, have some fun, and meet some locals – but I go armed with my phone so I can add anyone I meet to Facebook. If they're in my local area sooner or later these people are going to hit me up!

It's simply a numbers game – the more people you meet, the more successful your business is going to be. Also, the more people you meet, the more chance you have of meeting one of those people in there that can springboard you to a higher place – leading to our next strategy …

STRATEGY 2: Meet the RIGHT people

Knowing 100 people is great, but if you can know the RIGHT people it's going to count as a lot more than those 100. What I mean by that is if one of those 100 people happens to know lots of people in the area, then it's the JACKPOT. There's always that one person who just knows everyone; they've grown up in the area, they are very active in the community, they volunteer for all those things, they talk to everyone etc. If you can meet one of these people, you're laughing, because if they like you they'll promote you all over town! Alone they might be able to get you 5-15 people down to your bootcamp.

They could be members of the local community who see a lot of people, for example:

- Physio
- Local GP
- Hairdresser
- Beautician
- Chiropractor
- Nutritionist
- Café owner

I was doing a local Fun-Run with my bootcamp as one of our excursions. At the finish line, all the local businesses had tents set up, and I saw a physio there. I introduced myself, saying, 'Hey, I'm Jono. I'm a personal trainer, I run a bootcamp, and

I'm looking for a physio to connect with, because I want to send all my clients to the one place.' (I recommend having one physio who you can send your clients to, as it's more professional. You can say, 'Hey, I know a physio down the road, they're a good friend of mine. They'll give you a bit of a discount, and also gives me the rundown afterwards so we can tailor your training accordingly.')

So this physio and I connected, got talking for a few weeks, and came up with an arrangement: Once every 12 weeks (to coincide with my challenges) he'd send an email out to his list saying that his good friend, a PT (me) was offering one of his clients a free spot in a 12-Week Challenge. They had to email me to apply, and I offered everyone who didn't win two weeks for free.

Numerous advantages there. Number one is just list building; heaps of people would email me, I'd build my list and my database so that they could be clients down the track. Secondly, someone gets the free challenge, and my job is to convert that person to sign on again at the end of it, and those people who got the two week trial, same thing.

That worked really well, so I wanted to do the same thing with a chiro. I put it out to my friends, sent out some text messages, and made some Facebook posts asking if anyone had a recommendation. One of my clients had a chiropractor so I connected with that guy, got on really well, and went from there.

It wasn't a first-time thing – I'd tried many times to find people to connect with, and couldn't find a good match. It's important to be friends with that person so that you're both going to genuinely help each other out.

Another way I've connected with people is through local businesses. This is an interesting strategy – I actually only did it for 2-3 weeks then gave up, but I want to share it anyway because you might get some ideas. When I first starting running bootcamps, there was no such thing as Facebook ads, so I came up with this 'local business strategy'

I'd walk into a local business (e.g. café, hairdresser, beautician) and ask to speak to the manager. The person would look at me a bit scared – who's this guy? What's he complaining about? The manager would come out a bit defensive, but I'd just be super friendly. 'Hey, I'm Jono! I've just started up a bootcamp in the area, and I want to connect with as many local businesses as possible. I was thinking I could give all your clients a couple of free weeks of bootcamp.' I said I'd give them some fliers and a sheet where people could write their name, and at the end of the week I'd come to collect it. A lot of people told me to go away, but a lot of people went for it! At that age I was 25, a young go-getter. They saw I was out and giving it a go, so they decided to help me out.

Doing this took up a lot of my time; I picked four suburbs, 2-3 places in each, so I had 10-15 different places to visit every Friday. I was spending 10-20 minutes at each place to have a chat and build the relationship. I got a lot of leads, but often they didn't answer. After not getting any clients for that, I scrapped it.

However, one of the hairdressers I spoke to called me, saying, 'Not sure if you remember me, but I really want to train. I'm not happy with where my body's at, and you seem like a nice guy – can I come in and do your next 12-Week Challenge?' She became a client, liked it so much that she signed up for the year. I might have wasted some of my Fridays, but it gave me a client for 15 months – it's a pretty good deal, plus she referred a couple of her friends. They didn't sign up for the year, but one of them did three months, another did six.

There was one supplement store that was not even that close to where I trained, but I knew a person who worked there. She lived too far away to come to the sessions, but I invited her to join my Facebook Group instead. A couple of weeks later one of her friends moved to my area and was asking if anyone could recommend a PT, and my friend tagged me. At that stage I was getting out of the personal training business, focusing all on bootcamp, so I increased my rates. Personal training was $100, so $100 for 12 weeks (a one-on-one session with me, and unlimited access to bootcamp). I didn't want to do PT for less than $100, and I was at bootcamp anyway, so why not give them bootcamp for free? This person signed up, and it was by far the biggest sale I had ever made – $1200.

STRATEGY 3: ASSOCIATE with the right people

There's a saying that you're the sum of the four people you hang out with the most, and I really believe that. It might not be an exact science, but if your four best friends are millionaires, there's a pretty good chance you're going to be the 5th. It works the other way; if your four best friends are dropkicks, chances are you're going to be the 5th.

It's easy for a lot of personal trainers to realise this. Let's say you've got a family of five: mum, dad, and three kids aged 15, 19, and 21. The 19-year old girl comes to see you to get her fitness in order, but the rest of the family is super unhealthy. None of them exercise, and none of them eat healthy.

On the flipside, you've got a super healthy family of five. They eat really well, and they all do active things. You could give the exact same exercise and nutrition advice, but the one who's growing up in that unhealthy environment is going to be so much harder for them because they're going to be tempted with sweets around the place. They'll have to

and meet people. It's the easiest and cheapest way to get yourself out, and you might find you've got similar interests, or mutual friends, and that'll help you become friends.

You might not want to annoy your other friends by plugging business stuff, but if your friends aren't going to like it, who do you think will? Strangers? If there's one thing we've learned from social media, it's that you can't rely on the kindness of strangers; your friends are your best option in terms of liking and commenting and sharing. You're welcome to add us as a friend and look at what we post there. It's not only stuff about our business, it also general tips in life and things that we do, things we've found helpful or funny, and we might have a call to action at the end.

Action Tasks

1. Do something every week that ensures you are meeting locals!
2. Do something every week that ensures you are meeting the RIGHT people.
3. Hang out more with successful people – even if means paying!

Bootcamp A vs Bootcamp B

Instructor A doesn't go to any local networking opportunities, doesn't try and create a relationship with local 'heavy hitters', and doesn't surround themselves with other successful people.

Instructor B has a regular 'thing' they do every week where they connect with locals, they have a connection with at least one local 'heavy hitter' who constantly refers them clients (even though this took a while to get), and they surround themselves with other successful people – both in person and via reading books and listening to podcasts.

More information

This is the sort of content we cover in our Bootcamp CEC courses – to check them out, simply go to our website (www.fitnesseducationon line.com.au). Also make sure you join our community Facebook Group (www.facebook.com/groups/fitnesseducationonline) where we have over 8000 trainers from all over the world discussing these topics.

Books to read

Follow Me by Francesca Moi

Never Lose a Client Again

Retention is the most important topic when growing your bootcamp, because it's the quickest way to grow.

If you've got more clients leaving than you do coming in – you're never going to grow, no matter how many new clients you get.

Bootcamp A

Gets 20 participants registered for their first 12-Week Challenge. At the end of the 12 weeks, only 10 participants want to keep training (50% retention rate). Instructor A does some sales and marketing and gets another 10 new clients, so for their second bootcamp, Instructor A still only has 20 participants (10 old and 10 new).

Bootcamp B

Gets 20 participants registered for their first 12-Week Challenge. At the end of the 12 weeks, 18 participants want to keep training (90% retention rate). Instructor B does some sales and marketing and gets another 10 new clients, so for their second bootcamp, Instructor B now has 28 participants (18 old and 10 new)

Let's assume those stats say the same for the next bootcamp:

Bootcamp A (second challenge)

Still only has 20 participants registered. At the end of the 12 weeks, only 10 participants want to keep training (50% retention rate). Instructor A does some sales and marketing and gets another 10 new clients, so for their third bootcamp, Instructor A still only has 20 participants (10 old and 10 new).

Bootcamp B (second challenge)

Now has 28 participants registered. At the end of the 12 weeks, 25 participants want to keep training (90% retention rate). Instructor B does some sales and marketing and gets another 10 new clients, so for their third bootcamp, Instructor B now has 35 participants (25 old and 10 new).

You can see where this is going!

The other advantage with retention is it means that your marketing dollars are worth more. Let's say your 12-Week Challenge is worth $500 (so one client is worth $500), BUT if you know that there's a 90% chance that client's going to stay for 2-3 challenges, all of a sudden it's not just a $500 sale; it's a $1000 sale, or a $1500 sale.

This means that you can afford to put a bit more on marketing, because you know that one client is worth that much money.

Retention can depend on three things:

- How much your clients like YOU.
- How much your clients like EACH OTHER.
- How much FUN they have at the sessions.

How much your clients like YOU

This is important. I'm going to share a quote from Theodore Roosevelt that changed my life: 'Nobody cares how much you know until they know how much you care.'

Before I head this quote I was training to be the 'best-looking trainer' or the 'fittest trainer' or the 'strongest trainer', and my retention was rubbish. As soon as I changed my mindset to wanting to be the most 'supportive trainer' my retention went through the roof!

There's plenty of things you can do to make yourself more 'likable', and support is at the top at that list! The more supportive you can be, the more your clients will like you!

The other thing I recommend every trainer do is read *How to Win Friends and Influence People* by Dale Carnegie. It was published in 1936, and if you look at any successful person, it's always on their list of favourite books. He set out six points that I read it every day:

- Become genuinely interested in other people.
- Smile.
- Remember that a person's name is, to that person, the sweetest and most important sound in any language.
- Be a good listener. Encourage them to talk about themselves.
- Talk in terms of the other person's interests.
- Make the other person feel important – and do it sincerely.

The very first time I contact someone (usually when they enquire about the bootcamp) we chat for about 15-20 minutes about them and their goals – even though they haven't even signed up yet. If they then sign up, beautiful, I've already done the goal-setting session. If they don't sign up, that's okay, I've had a really good conversation with them and chances are they're going to come back later.

Once they've signed up I add them on Facebook, add them to my Facebook group, and like a few of their photos. I also take a quick video on my phone of me welcoming them to the program and text it to them where I say, 'Hi, [insert name]! Jono here from Outdoor Bootcamp, super excited that you're getting started, look forward to meeting you, have a good one. Just wanted to take a video so you can put a name to a face!'

I then stay in touch with them until bootcamp starts. A week beforehand I'll send a text and say, 'Hi, [insert first name], we kick off bootcamp next week, is everything good to go on your end?' I do the same thing before their first session saying, 'Hi, [insert first name], we kick off bootcamp tomorrow, is everything good to go on your end?'

Those points there will get you in good stead. I believe that 50% of retention is done before you even meet the client, so:

» The first phone call.
» The video text message straight after.
» The Facebook friendship.
» The two follow-up texts before their first session.

If you do those things there you're off to a good start.

Next, I'd probably say 40% of retention comes down to their first week. In that first week you've got to knock their socks off – training wise *and* support wise!

Training-wise – you want to run your most fun, engaging sessions that are catered for all levels. This will clients the opportunity to keep up, meet others in the group, and have fun.

Support-wise – you obviously need to be supportive during the session (use Dale Carnegie's strategies) and there's two key text messages to send during the week. The first should come after their first session (that day if it's an AM session, or the next day if it's a PM session). It should read, 'Hey, [insert first name], how are you? Awesome to meet you this morning, just wanted to text and see how you're enjoying bootcamp, how's the body holding up?' The second message comes after their first week, saying, 'Hey, [insert first name], how are you? Just wanted to text and see how you enjoyed your first week at bootcamp? Body feeling ok?'

From there it's just consistency; keep in touch with them throughout the challenge every week, and every couple of weeks send a text message, and make sure you're speaking to them during the session. If you can do those things there, you're going to become very likeable and your retention is going to go through the roof.

How much your clients like EACH OTHER

This is just as important as the first point because it's all well and good if a client likes you, but if they hate each other they are not coming back, no matter how charming you are! What's important here is to realise that it is the trainer's responsibility to get their clients to like each other.

It's a learned skill. You've got to read all the books on group dynamics and group bonding, but even then you can't *make* someone like someone else. You *can* create and foster an environment that makes it easier for people to meet each other and get to know each other, or worst-case scenario, not hate each other!

A couple things you can do as the trainer

- Get to each session at least half an hour early. Spend 15 minutes setting up and preparing for the session, and then 15 minutes working on 'group bonding'. By the time people start coming in, you're already set up and are waiting for your clients to arrive. I set up the seating arrangements so anyone who comes early is forced to sit next to someone else – not just stand in the corner on their phone. This is very important before training; I want to get as much chatter as possible, and encourage people to come down and talk to each other before training.
- Start with a game. My warm up is 10mins: a five minute functional warmup, and then a five minute game. The game is purely to get people bonding/talking to each other/meeting each other. This is key at the START of the session because it sets the tone for the rest of the session.
- Always do something during the session that encourages group interaction. So many different options: partner workouts, partner drills, partner stretches, team drills, boxing – it's endless!
- After the session I encourage people to hang around and just chat. I take my time packing up and make sure everyone knows I'm in no rush to get out of there, so they can chat as long as they like!
- Make sure you do excursions, it gets people to talk/interact/mingle outside of training! That makes a BIG difference! You go from training at the same place to hanging out socially! What's important with these excursions is that are

things that encourage people to bond. You don't just want to have an awkward party where no one talks to anyone new. You need to make sure the activity is interactive (e.g. rock climbing, outrigger canoeing, etc.).

How much FUN they are having

It's all well and good if your clients like you and each other, but if your workouts are boring, they're going to stop coming.

What's fun for one person might not be fun for another, so what's key is to find what fun is for your clientele and encourage more of it!

FAQ

'How can I keep people interested when situations change, they have a new timetable, they move out of the area, or winter sport starts?'

If you've done a good enough job they're still going to come back. If someone leaves our bootcamp because they got a new a job and now need to leave earlier, we haven't done a good enough job of making bootcamp the most important thing in these people's lives.

If we did a good enough job they wouldn't have taken the new job because they knew they would miss bootcamp. They can get a new job anywhere, but my bootcamp is a once in a lifetime opportunity.

Retention is 110% your responsibility. Every single person who doesn't sign back up happens because you didn't hit 3/3 of those things.

Action Tasks

1. Do something every week to make you more likable.
2. Do something every week that shows your clients you're supporting them.
3. Do something every week that is bringing your clients closer together.
4. Do something every session to make it fun!

Bootcamp A vs Bootcamp B

Instructor A doesn't study anything on how to be more 'likable'; they just think if they be themselves that's enough. They don't do anything to foster group dynamics, they simply think running the bootcamp, and doing the odd partner drill is enough. They don't do anything to make the activity more fun, they think because it's exercise it doesn't have to be fun.

Instructor B continually studies how to be 'likable' and is always doing extras to show their clients how much they care about them. They constantly study group dynamics and always come up with ways to bring the group closer to together. They are always looking for fun things to do or little ways to make the sessions more fun for participants.

More information

This is the sort of content we cover in our Bootcamp CEC courses – to check them out, simply go to our website (www.fitnesseducationon line.com.au). Also make sure you join our community Facebook Group (www.facebook.com/groups/fitnesseducationonline) where we have over 8000 trainers from all over the world discussing these topics.

Books to read

How to Win Friends and Influence People by Dale Carnegie

Raving Fans by Ken Blanchard

How to Turn Your Clients into Your No-Commission Sales Team

I love referrals for two major reasons:

1. They're cost effective, because they cost nothing.
2. They are the easiest sales to make, because one of their trusted friends has already vouched for you!

A common mistake that trainers make is that they think as long as they do a good job, people are going to refer their friends, and there is some truth in that. However, it's not a system – you can't just turn the tap on, do a really good job this weekend, and expect people will come down. There is a way you *can* turn the tap on, and that's the 'Bring a Friend Week'. I've got this down to a science, so let me break it down for you!

When I run a 12-Week Challenge, I will always do my 'Bring a Friend Week' in Week 6, the halfway point, the reason being is if those friends enjoy training with me, I allow them to sign up for a little 6-Week Challenge for weeks 7-12.It works really well because at that stage numbers may start to drop a little bit, so you can handle the extras with no dramas. You can also hold it in Week 12 because that way if they enjoy it, the next challenge begins the following week.

What's important with 'Bring a Friend Week' is that it's done properly, because I've run bad ones before and no friends have come down. Now I've got it perfect and it works every time. There hasn't been a time where I haven't been able to get a whole heap of friends to come down, and the majority of those friends sign up.

It's a 5-step process:

Step 1: The Week

This week has to be the best week of training in the whole challenge. I save all my best games, all my best drills, and my most fun workouts for Week 6 (I also do some of them in Week 1). The mistake I used to make was not planning that workout for the friends, instead just planning it for the group, so it's been really hard, intense, and not that fun. The friends haven't been able to keep up, or they haven't had fun.

I also make sure I do an excursion that week. On the weekend we do something fun (stand-up paddleboarding, rock climbing, pole dancing), so by the end of that week, the friends think the bootcamp is awesome. Every single session has been fun and interactive, I've met people who have kept up, and they come with us on the weekend.

Step 2: Promotion

It's all well and good to make it your most fun week, but if no one's down there, what's the point? It's essential that you promote it properly. When I first started running 'Bring a Friend Week', I just let people know the week before. Not many people brought friends.

I had to think about what I could do to get as many people down as possible, and the first thing I did was put together a priority pass.

BRING A FRIEND PRIORITY PASS

NAME:

PHONE NUMBER:

EMAIL ADDRESS:

FRIEND REFERRED BY:

WHICH SESSION(S) ARE YOU LOOKING TO ATTEND:

PLEASE ANSWER THE FOLLOWING QUESTIONS

1.	Has your doctor ever told you that you have a heart condition or have you ever suffered a stroke?	Yes	No
2.	Do you ever experience unexplained pains in your chest at rest or during physical activity/exercise?	Yes	No
3.	Do you ever feel faint or have spells of dizziness during physical activity/exercise that causes you to lose balance?	Yes	No
4.	Have you had an asthma attack requiring immediate medical attention at any time over the last 12 months?	Yes	No
5.	If you have diabetes (type I or type II) have you had trouble controlling your blood glucose in the last 3 months?	Yes	No
6.	Do you have any diagnosed muscle, bone or joint problems that you have been told could be made worse by participating in physical activity/exercise?	Yes	No
7.	Do you have any other medical condition(s) that may make it dangerous for you to participate in physical activity/exercise?	Yes	No

Thank you

Jonathon Petrohilos
jono@outdoorbootcamp.com.au
0412 758 031

'Hey, Maria, what's up? I know we spoke a couple of weeks ago when you weren't quite ready to do the challenge, just letting you know I'm doing a free week next week. Did you want to come down?'

Who's going to say no to that?

Step 3: Lead generation

Part of the reason why I do this priority pass is that a lot of people say their friend is going to come down, but that friend doesn't end up coming. If 20 people have said they're bringing a friend, chances are it's going to be more like 10-15 people who come down. But I don't wait to waste the opportunity those 5-10 people offer; I've got their name, number, and email. I'm still going to give them a call, send them a text message, add them to my community Facebook Group, to my email list, and to my text message list, because they could be a client further down the line. Even if their friend stops training with me, I can still send out an email with a special offer, or when they're ready to train then we can chat.

Step 4: Lead nurturing

Once I get these priority passes, I treat the friend like I would an actual client. I use the exact same retention process.

» The 15-20min welcome call.
» Add to Facebook, Facebook Group, video text.
» Text them before their first session.
» Send them a text after their first session.

Step 5: The Sale

The 'friend' isn't necessarily going to text you and say they want to join, so you always need to ask! When you send the end of week text, tell them about the 6-Week Challenge and offer a discount.

If you can follow these steps, you're going to get a whole heap of people down at the training, you're going to convert them into clients, and it's going to grow your business – all for free.

Once you've got it down-pat you can spend a few dollars to make it even more effective –I get so many people coming down for this week that I need to bring another trainer in. I've had times where I get 20 people per session and can run them on my own, but every single one of them wants to bring a friend so I have to hire another trainer to come down to take the other 20.

FAQ

'Do you give kickbacks? So if a client refers a friend, do you give the client a free week, or a free month?

We don't want people to refer friends so they get money. We want someone to refer a friend because they love the experience with me, and they genuinely want to share it around. We do send them a personalised thank you via text. We also send them a voucher equivalent to one week of training, so they pretty much do get a week free of training, but we don't tell them that beforehand. We don't do referral draws for the same reason.

'Can you do all this online?'

Yes, you can. We use this strategy to grow our community Facebook Group. Tell your friends in the group to refer a friend into the group, get them to send you a message with their details, and then you'll do an online draw – every friend you refer, you go into the draw to win a free 12-Week Online Program.

Action Tasks

1. Set up your 'Bring a Friend Week'. Plan EVERYTHING about it – promotion and activities!

Bootcamp A vs Bootcamp B

Instructor A doesn't actively promote referrals. Every now and then they'll do a 'Bring a Friend Week', but they don't really promote it or do anything different during the week. Instructor A doesn't get many referrals.

Instructor B already has their 'Bring a Friend Week' planned, they know exactly what week it is, exactly what activities they are doing, and exactly how they are going to promote it. They always get plenty of people coming down, and get new clients from it every time!

More information

This is the sort of content we cover in our Bootcamp CEC courses – to check them out, simply go to our website (www.fitnesseducationon line.com.au). Also make sure you join our community Facebook Group (www.facebook.com/groups/fitnesseducationonline) where we have over 8000 trainers from all over the world discussing these topics.

Books to read

The Referral of a Lifetime by Tim Templeton.

Endless Referrals by Bob Burg.

The One-Percenters Make All the Difference

You're not judged on your workouts. You can get two trainers to give the same group of clients the exact same workout, but these clients might like one trainer more than the other because the trainer is a better instructor because of 'one-percenters'.

The advantage of being a good instructor is that another trainer can come up with a creative workout, but you can take that workout, put your spin on it, and use your skills to make it better.

If a trainer is not a good instructor, they can't do that. They may be able to get on YouTube and get a workout, but if they can't get their participants to go to that workout, it's worthless. That's why it's so important to be a good instructor and do these little one-percenters here.

I'm going to cover three things in this section:

- Explanations or instructions.
- How to scale.
- Motivation and energy.

Explanations and instructions

How do you explain a workout? That can make or break the workout. No one wants to go to a workout and not know what they're doing, or if they're doing it right, or how many reps they're doing, so you need to explain it properly. It should not be a riddle!

Don't over-explain either. Let's just take an exercise like a squat. Every single trainer could probably spend an hour explaining how to do a squat in the best way, but no one's going to come to a bootcamp to hear you talk about a squat for an hour. It needs to be clear and concise.

Cater to the different learning styles; auditory, visually, or kinesthetically. Write the workout on a whiteboard so the visual people can see it. Then explain it so the auditory people can hear it. Then demonstrate it so the visual people see you do it. Lastly, get the participants to practice it so the kinesthetic people can do it. You cover all bases!

Make sure everyone can see and hear you. You don't want to have your back to anyone (so no circles around you). If you've got a stage step up on that so you're easier to see and you're in that dominant position. If you're outside, be aware of the wind and sun. Cover as much of it as possible in the warmup so there's less you need to explain in the workout.

How to scale

Now you want to scale the 'exercise' and the 'workout'. To scale an exercise is pretty basic. Using squats as an example again – get all your participants to do squats for a minute. If they are all at different levels, one person may find squatting for a minute not challenging enough, and another may find it too challenging. You'll want some different options, so if squatting for a minute is too difficult, just do a half squat. If squatting for a minute is too easy, do squat jumps! It's then your job as the trainer to walk around and make sure everyone's doing it at their own level in a safe and effective way.

We'll talk a little bit about scaling the whole workout later, but what's important as an instructor is you can't have workouts where someone's coming first and someone's coming last. Let's say participants need to finish as quick as they can, and the quickest person finishes in 20 minutes and the slowest person finishes in 30 minutes. That's not a good workout because

» the quickest person is doing less work than the slowest person. If anything, the fittest person should be doing more work. They should be going for 30 minutes, and the beginner should be going for 20 minutes.
» if that advanced person finishes the workout in 20 minutes, what do they do? Sit around and wait for everyone else? That's boring. Sooner or later, they're going to get sick of that.
» the person who came last is going to feel like CRAP! They are not going back either because they think the bootcamp is too hard for them!

I'll go through some tips when we're talking about workouts, but you've got a few basic options.

- Time-based (e.g. circuit, AMRAP, HIIT).
- First to finish (once the first person finishes the workout, everyone else can stop).

Motivation and energy

The most important part of being a good instructor is the motivation and the energy, because if you're a half-decent trainer you can probably explain things all right and scale things, but what's going to make the biggest difference is the motivation and the energy. You may think you're in the training business, but we're in the entertainment business. People aren't going to come to train if it's boring, because there's so many other fun things to do in life. We need to make our bootcamp fun.

There are many different ways you can provide motivation and energy:

- *Music* – It makes your session more motivating. You can work out in dead quiet, but that's pretty boring. If you can add some motivating music, that's going to add so much more to your session.
- *Voice* – Who would you rather train with? Someone who has a boring, monotone voice, or someone who sounds a lot more exciting?
- *Phone timer* – You don't want to sit around looking at your stopwatch because that takes you out of your session. You want all that automated so you can walk around the room and provide the motivation, support, and the technical advice.
- *One-on-one* – It's not all about you standing up

the front yelling fitness clichés. It's better if you walk around to every single person, stay with them for a bit, encourage them by name, and help them count out a few reps. You can see there how that's way more motivating.

» *Small space* – Get everyone in a small space and pair them up. Even if it's not a part of the workout, I ideally want two lines of people facing a partner. I want everyone to feel like there's someone in front of them and someone to either side of them, so you're not just sitting alone in the corner doing the workout on your own.

» *Interval break* – If it's a workout like an AMRAP, which is 20 minutes of the same thing over and over again, I'll add in a timer for every two minutes where participants do 20 star jumps. That gives them a bit of a break, adds an interval, and adds some energy to it!

» *Shoulder tap* – At random intervals I tap someone on the shoulder and get them to do 20 battle rope slams, or 10 medicine ball slams, or whatever it may be. It adds some energy to the workout because participants have always got to look over their shoulder for you.

Action Tasks

1. Always think about the most effective way you can explain a workout.
2. Always think of different ways you can scale a workout/exercise.
3. Always think of different ways you can add motivation and energy to your workout.

Bootcamp A vs Bootcamp B

Instructor A can come up with a really creative, effective workout, but doesn't put much effort into explaining it, so a lot of people get confused. Instructor A doesn't put a heap of motivation and energy into the session; they may walk around a little bit and give some general encouragement, but not by their name.

Instructor B can come up with a really creative, effective workout, but they can make even an average workout a lot more fun because they explain it effectively, give scalable options for everyone, and provide so much motivation and energy that the participants have fun no matter what they do!

More information

This is the sort of content we cover in our Bootcamp and Functional Training CEC courses – to check them out, simply go to our website (www.fitnesseducationonline.com.au). Also make sure you join our community Facebook Group (www.facebook.com/groups/fitnesseducationonline) where we have over 8000 trainers from all over the world discussing these topics.

Equipment Myths

I get it all the time, people saying, 'I want to start a bootcamp, I'm going to spend $1000 on equipment – what should I get?' I recommend people get their equipment over a year. If you're running a 12-Week Challenge, you're going to run four of them throughout the year, and every challenge you're going to spend $300. If you do it like this, you're going to get a lot more clients because your sessions are going to more varied. It's not like you're getting all this equipment at the start, outlaying $1000 and then you're stressed – all you need to do is outlay $300, you can do a lot of varied workouts for this amount, and then for the next challenge you get a new lot of equipment that adds more variety.

Not only is it cost-effective, it's also time-efficient, because packing and unpacking all that equipment takes a long time! If you're running an hour session, it might take you 15 minutes to pack your car from your garage. You might then have to get to training 15 minutes early to unpack your car and setting up, then after your session you're going to have to spend another 15 minutes putting it all back in your car, then more time getting it from your car to your garage.

This book is meant to teach you how to make 6-figures a year, working 60mins a day, so if you're spending 60mins just packing your car, you're in trouble! It also helps you be space-efficient. I drive a Honda Civic, and I can only fit so much equipment in it, so I've got to make sure it doesn't take up a lot of space.

It's important that the equipment is varied; there's no point in getting a piece of equipment if you're only going to do one exercise on it. Your goal is to get equipment where you can do a lot of different effective exercises on it, one that doesn't take up a lot of space, time, and doesn't cost a lot.

Let's assume you're getting 18 people to your sessions.

Stage 1: $300

» *Bodyweight – free!*

The first thing is bodyweight, which costs you absolutely nothing. I recommend that you get really good with bodyweight exercise workouts and drills. All over YouTube are variations of basic bodyweight exercises, like squats and lunges. It's important to get very good at them, because that's how you become a good trainer. The less equipment you have, the more imaginative you can get, and the better you can get as a trainer.

» *Surroundings – free!*

From there, you want to have a look at your surroundings. The two easiest things are walls and benches, because if you've got a wall you can do things like wall squats and holes, and benches are good for dips and step-ups.

I recommend having a specific beach session, a specific hill session, and a specific stair session. Just by changing the location, you get variety for free.

» *Skipping ropes and ladders – $40*

You can get skipping ropes for $2 from Kmart. Get at least 9 or 10 skipping; that way, if you've got 18-20 people, you've got a skipping rope between two and heaps of drills you can do. I also recommend an agility ladder, which is going to cost you $20, but you can fit at least 10 people on there, too.

If you were starting off with just $40, you've got the bodyweight, you've got the surroundings, your different locations, a heap of skipping ropes, and an agility ladder.

» *Boxing Gear – $200-$300*

Optional, but recommended because it's an awesome workout, it's a partner workout, and it's different. Boxing is a completely different form of training to the previous ones, and so varied. There are many different ways you can do boxing sessions, and you basically just need gloves and focus pads. When starting off, ask participants to bring their own gloves (especially for hygiene reasons). You might bring a couple of spare pairs in case someone forgets theirs.

You provide the focus pads, and you only need one between two. You can get them for $20-$30, sometimes in a package with gloves. You can keep the pads and sell the gloves to your clients. Get 9-10 pairs of gloves and pads for about $200-$300.

» *Battle rope – $50*

Also optional, but a great one. You can get a battle rope on eBay for about $50. I think that's worth it, as you only need one for your whole group. This works well for the people who struggle to run, skip, or jump, because the battle rope is an amazing cardio drill.

To summarise, get really good at your bodyweight exercises. See if there's some benches and walls around where you're training so you can add some more variety. Make sure you've got space where you can do the odd session where there's some hills and stairs and a beach. Get some ladders and skipping ropes. Optional equipment is focus pads and gloves, and a battle rope.

Stage 2: $300

» *Suspension trainer (TRX), and resistance bands – ($10-$30)*

The advantage to these is they're so light and portable, like the ladder and the skipping rope. I'll take the suspension trainer over anything else because it's got exercise variety, and unlike kettlebells, I can easily fit 6 TRXs in my bag! It also helps that the exercise will be the same with everyone who tries it, whereas with a kettlebell you'd need to switch weights. It adds a whole other dynamic. If you went through your first 12-Week Challenge with just the bodyweight stuff and the ladder, buying the bands and the suspension trainers takes you to a whole new level.

Stage 3: $300

» *Kettlebells – $50*

This is when you bring some of the weighted stuff. You can choose either a kettlebell or a medicine ball, whatever works better. You're going to get about six kettlebells, and at $50 each there's your $300. In terms of weights, I recommend 3x8kg, and 3x12kg. If you've got someone who's too strong for a 12kg, they do a single arm kettlebell swing. If someone thinks 8kgs is too heavy, do bodyweight squats instead of kettlebell squats.

The reason I like kettlebells and the med balls is that you can add them to any exercise. You can add weight to your squats, lunges, and bridges, but they also add a ballistic side; you've got the kettlebell swing and its variations, the med ball slam and throw variations.

Stage 4: $300

If you got kettlebells in Stage 3, it's time to get the med balls now.

After a year, and $1200, you've now got six kettlebells, six med balls, a battle rope, six suspension trainers, six resistance bands, nine skipping ropes, nine ladders, all your boxing stuff, and your bodyweight stuff – you'll be unstoppable.

FAQ

'What if I have nowhere to hang a TRX?'

We will only run a bootcamp if there's somewhere we can hang a TRX, as we use them nearly every session.

'Jono/Travis, what if your weights get too easy for advanced clients, and you need to provide heavier ones?'

90% of that has nothing to do with weights. We look at our equipment we've got and figure out the most effective workouts we can do. If the kettlebell is too light, do a single arm kettlebell, a single arm rack position squat, etc.

It comes down to your niche, as well. Ideally, you're not going to be training an absolute beginner old lady alongside a body builder in the one bootcamp. You're going to have it niched; mums, all-women, or bodybuilders, so your weight hangs around that there. Worst-case scenario, just get one heavier one, a 16kg kettlebell.

Action Tasks

1. Get good at bodyweight workouts.
2. Get good at using your surroundings.
3. Get good at using skipping ropes/ladders.
4. Get trained in boxing, and then buy some gear.
5. Get trained in suspension, bands, kettlebells, med balls, battle ropes, and get some gear.

Bootcamp A vs Bootcamp B

Instructor A has a heap of equipment. They spend 30mins setting up the session and 30mins packing up, so they don't have the time to liaise with clients before/after.

They currently don't have a big client-base because they haven't been doing any paid marketing (they are short on cash after buying all the equipment). Their workouts/ exercises also aren't that varied because they haven't been to many continuing education courses (also because they are short of money).

Instructor B doesn't have a lot of equipment, but has enough for plenty of variety because they know how to use the equipment effectively. This is because Instructor B has invested heavily on upskilling courses.

Instructor B gets on really well with their clients because they hang around with them for 15mins before every session (because it only takes 15mins to set up). Instructor B is also very busy at the moment because the money they saved on buying a heap of equipment is spent on advertising. Now that Instructor B is doing well financially, they are going to invest in more equipment.

More information

This is the sort of content we cover in our Bootcamp and Functional Training CEC courses – to check them out, simply go to our website (www.fitnesseducationonline.com.au). Also make sure you join our community Facebook Group (www.facebook.com/groups/fitnesseducationonline) where we have over 8000 trainers from all over the world discussing these topics.

How to Create Unlimited Bootcamp Workouts

You can have the best sales strategies, the best marketing, the fanciest website, all these retention and referral strategies, but if your workouts are boring nobody's coming back. They're not even going to finish the challenge.

With workouts, I look at three things your bootcamp workout is meant to be: safe, fun, and effective. If you can hit all three of those things, your clients are coming back. And they're pretty straightforward, right? If the workout's dangerous, people are going to get injured. It's not fun, it's going to be boring and people aren't going to come back. If it's not effective enough to get physical results, they're probably going to give up.

My workouts are broken down into three different parts: full bootcamp workouts, bootcamp games, and bootcamp drills. In this chapter I'm going to speak mainly about the full bootcamp workouts, but I want to touch on the other two.

Bootcamp games

I always do a 10-minute warmup for every bootcamp session. This includes a 5-minute functional warmup and a 5-minute fitness game. Come up with 12 really good fitness games and play one a week. See table below:

1	Numbers	Numbers	Numbers	Boxing	Boxing	Numbers
2	SPR	SPR	SPR	Boxing	Boxing	SPR
3	Towel Circle	Towel Circle	Towel Circl	Boxing	Boxing	Towel Circle
4	Hills Hollows	Hills Hollows	Hills Hollows	Boxing	Boxing	Hills Hollows
5	Tunnel	Tunnel	Tunnel	Boxing	Boxing	Tunnel
6	Rob the nest	Rob the nest	Rob the nest	Boxing	Boxing	Rob the nest
7	5 pass	5 pass	5 pass	Boxing	Boxing	5 pass
8	Card Game	Card Game	Card Game	Boxing	Boxing	Card Game
9	Directions	Directions	Directions	Boxing	Boxing	Directions
10	Noodle tag	Noodle tag	Noodle tag	Boxing	Boxing	Noodle tag
11	Actions game	Actions game	Actions game	Boxing	Boxing	Actions game
12	Cat and mouse	Cat and mouse	Cat and mouse	Boxing	Boxing	Cat and mouse

You get a free copy if you're in our Facebook Group. If you don't have a copy, just make a post on the Facebook Group or send me a PM, and I'll get you the copy. I used to try and play a different game every single session, and it was just too hard and confusing.

The advantage of playing the same game every day for a week is that you can start simple, then build it up.

You will also be teaching it several times to people who

come along to sessions later in the week.

Bootcamp drills

These 5-10 minute drill are done at the end of the session, before your five minutes of stretching. The finisher is always something fun or partner-based.

The meat of the workout is the hard part, and that may not always be super engaging, so start and end the sessions with something more fun.

Come up with 12 really good finishers, a couple of partner ones, and couple of drills to music.

These are my favourite ones; you do the Bring Sally Up, the Uptown Funk, the Nutbush Plank, the Plank Charger, Who Let the Dogs Out, Down ... there's plenty of them.

You get these for free if you're in the Facebook group, so if you don't have them, just hit me up.

Full bootcamp workouts

I promise that you can come up with unlimited bootcamp workouts.

So, there's the actual workout style, and then there's the exercises. I'll start with the style and then I'll get to the exercises.

What I recommend in a 12-Week Challenge is to run four bootcamp sessions, two boxing sessions.

Have enough to last you six weeks without repeating, so

you'll basically need 24 bootcamp workouts, and 12 boxing workots.

See the table below.

1	54321	AMRAP	Accumulator	Boxing 1	Boxing 2	Matrix
2	HIIT	Circuit	Leg day	Boxing 3	Boxing 4	Stairs
3	Arm Day	Super Set	10 to 1	Boxing 5	Boxing 6	Beach
4	Phone Number	100 Club	12 Cones	Boxing 7	Boxing 8	Excursion 1
5	Games Day	Trapp	Holiday	Boxing 9	Boxing 10	Traditional
6	Celebrity Day	3x3, 2x2, 1x1	Accumulating AMRAP	Boxing 11	Boxing 12	Tabata
7				Boxing 2	Boxing 1	
8				Boxing 4	Boxing 3	
9				Boxing 6	Boxing 5	
10				Boxing 8	Boxing 7	
11				Boxing 10	Boxing 9	
12				Boxing 12	Boxing 11	

The advantage to varying up the style is that I could just do the exact same exercises. One day I could say, 'Here are the six different exercises we're going to do, and today they'll be a circuit. We're going to do a minute on each station, four times through.'

The next day you say, 'Same exercise, but now it's an AMRAP. We're going to do 24 reps of these six different exercises, and we're going to do it as many times as we can in 24 minutes. Let's see how many times we can get through.'

Essentially the exact same workout, but it feels a bit different because one's a time-based one, one's a rep-based one.

You could then do it as an accumulator the next day. Those same six exercises, but in the first round they do three reps of everything, then six, then nine, and keep going until the timer ends.

You could then bring in those automated timer add-ons I mentioned earlier, where every two minutes my timer goes off and they do 20 star jumps before continuing on.

In the accumulator I make them do a 10m shuttle run. Just by adding those little differences there, it completely changes the workout.

Don't get me wrong, I'm not saying do the exact same exercises. I'm going to show you how to come up with different ones, but I just want you to get your head around how if you can come up with those 24 different workout styles, it's going to be a lot easier.

I suggest you balance it out and order it a bit. The way I order it is I start with the functional exercises.

Depending on who you speak to, they're going to tell you different things about functional exercises, but the common thing is the functional exercises are squat, lunge, hinge, push, pull.

Some people might tell you there's got to be a rotation there, and some people might say there's going to be a gait in there.

What I recommend to start with, even just bodyweight-wise, is to come up with all those different variations.

How many bodyweight squat variations are there?

How many bodyweight lunge variations can I come up with?

How much bodyweight hinges?

How many pushes and pulls?

Rotations and gaits?

Squat	**Lunge**	**Push**	**Pull**	**Hinge**
Squat	Lunge			
Squat Jump	Side Lunge			
Squat Hold	Curtsy Lunge			
Squat Pulse	Alternate Lunge			
Side Squat	Static Lunge			
Walking Squat	Jumping Lunge			
Pistol Squat	Walking Lunge			
Wall Sit	Lunge and Kick			

Write up a different list to that. Once you've got that, do the same thing with equipment.

With a kettlebell, what are the different squat variations can I do?

And with lunges?

Same thing with the hinge, the push, etc.

Then repeat with every functional exercise.

Squat	Lunge	Push	Pull	Hinge
Goblet Squat				
Rack Squat				
Squat and Press				
Cossack Squat				
Overhead Squat				
Waiters Squat				
Bottoms Up Squat				

Then do the same thing with different bits of equipment. With a med ball, what are the different functional exercises? With a TRX what can I do? With a resistance band what can I do? Once you've got all those different variations there, then you can just plug it in and say, 'All right, this week I'm going to do a circuit on Monday with only a kettlebell, so all my exercises are going to be the bodyweight or the kettlebell. The next day I'm going to do an AMRAP with a medicine ball. The next day I'm going to bring a TRX down.' You can mix and match like that.

The same thing with the exercises. You could do an AMRAP every single session, but you bring a different bit of equipment down every day so it feels like a different workout. But I'm recommending changing those exercises and changing the workouts, as well, so you literally just come up with unlimited variations. Add on top of that the different games and drills you've got, it's just endless. You're never going to do the exact same workout again, not even close to it.

If you've got enough for six weeks of workouts, repeat them. You could repeat those exact same workouts, because it's been six weeks since people have done it so they've forgotten about it, or they want to do it again to test their fitness. Make it slightly different; instead of doing that AMRAP with a kettlebell, now you're doing it with a med ball.

If you use those functional exercises you're usually in a pretty good position, but it's also important to focus on three things that I consider: different chains, different planes, and different positions.

» *Chains*

The common issue you see with bootcamp instructors is that they overdo the anterior chain, and underdo the posterior chain. They'll do their squats, their lunges, and their pushups because it's so easy in bootcamp, but they'll skip the pull and hinge because they don't have the equipment, or it's harder to do those exercises. It's very important not to skip those ones. That's why I love TRXs and kettlebells, because they're so good for both.

» *Planes*

You've got three different planes: frontal, sagittal, and transverse. If you're not too sure about those, you can Google them. What we find in bootcamp and in the gym is a lot of people overdo the sagittal plane; the squats, lunges, pushups, pulls, the hinges. If you're not careful or creative, all those functional movements can be done just in the sagittal plan – and that's an issue.

I look at my planned workout check what plane every exercise is in. Is there at least one transverse plane exercise in there? If there's not, how can I add it in? Am I going to bring a couple of bands down and do some of my wood chopper variations, or anti-rotation variations? Am I going to change the med ball slams? Do I do med ball rainbow slams so I'm rotating there? Or am I going to add a twist to my lunge?

Same thing with the frontal plane. If everything's in the sagittal plane, how am I going to change these squats? I'm going to change it to a squat and a walk to the side? Am I going to put some booty bands on? Instead of doing my lunge am I going to do a curtsey lunge? Or am I going to do a side lunge?

Different positions

Your options include:

- » Standing
- » Seated
- » Kneeling
- » Prone
- » Supine

Action Tasks

1. Come up with six weeks of different workouts

Bootcamp A vs Bootcamp B

Instructor A just does a Circuit or Tabata every session.

Instructor B has six weeks of completely different workouts styles.

More information

This is the sort of content we cover in our Bootcamp and Functional Training CEC courses – to check them out, simply go to our website (www.fitnesseducationonline.com.au). Also make sure you join our community Facebook Group (www.facebook.com/groups/fitnesseducationonline) where we have over 8000 trainers from all over the world discussing these topics.

Make Money While You Sleep

There's two ways you can do this:

- Hire another trainer
- Get online

My advice is to start looking for a trainer now, because if you ever want to take a holiday, or a day off, need a sick day or a personal day, or actually want to do something outside of work, you need to have another trainer working for you as a backup. If you do this properly, you can make money while you sleep.

If, for example, you're running a bootcamp with 20 participants (all paying $50 per week), you're making $1000 per week. If you want to take a week off and go to Thailand to relax, great – hire another trainer to run your sessions, paying them $50 a session (if you're running six sessions a week, that totals $300 to the trainer). You're still making $700 a week kicking back on the beach in Thailand!

But you need to find that person early and build them up! Even just starting off with one session a week while you're there, because if you decide to go on holidays next month, it's going to be near impossible to find a trainer up to the standard you want to run your sessions while you're gone. If you've had a trainer working under you for the last few weeks/months and you trust them – then you can take your holiday!

There are other advantages to having a backup trainer.

Handle more clients

I discussed this one in an earlier chapter. If you get a sudden influx of new clients ('Bring a Friend Week', or just new people signing up), you just can't give everyone the support they need.

People might start to leave if they think they aren't getting your full attention, and there is nothing more frustrating when that happens because you know how hard it is to get your numbers up that high, and then go back down. If you had another trainer there, you can BOTH handle 15-20 people each, so you can have 30-40 people down to your session and comfortably give them the support they need!

Session variety

Working solo, you've got to be so creative to keep your sessions fresh. If you've got another trainer there, you can leverage off their creativity.

Let your trainer run one session per week on their own; they can get creative, and that's one less session you need to worry about. You might still go there and help out with technique or do the support, but you don't need to worry about the variety.

Expansion

If you ever want to expand your bootcamps out to another area, you would be able to split your time between the two, whilst your trainer would run the other.

When I first started running a bootcamp it was small, only 15-20 people registered. I had 5-10 people per session, so I didn't need another trainer. But I actually hired two trainers; one to run my Monday session, and one to run my Tuesday session.

The reasons I hired straight away was that

» I couldn't do Monday morning, I was still working at the gym and there was one slot that I couldn't get off. I needed to stay at the gym for another month or two before leaving.

» I had a good friend who was a really, really good trainer, and I wanted them to run a session so my clients would get to experience some variety. I still came down to training to help out, but it was her session.

I also did it a little bit out of fear, because I wanted to take the pressure off me. I wasn't confident enough to run six sessions a week – I didn't think I had the workout variety. The best thing was that, once I got busier, I already had the team. Once I was getting 40 people down per session, it was very easy for me just to say, 'Monday trainer – can you also do Wednesday and Friday? Tuesday Trainer – can you also do Thursday?'

It was such an easy transition. I didn't need to sweat about finding a trainer to help me because I already had two who I knew were good, and had been working with me for six months!

FAQ

'Jono/Travis, I've been looking, but I haven't found anyone for my team. How do I find good trainers?'

Look harder; we've never had a drama hiring trainers, because we've just always been looking. When we were working at the gym, we made sure that we met every single trainer who worked there. Even before we were running bootcamp, we wanted a connection with every single one of them, because you never know when you're going to need it. We've always met trainers when we've done courses, and we go to all the conventions and conferences, and we make sure that we add people on Facebook. When we go to different gyms, we make sure that we speak to the trainers and get to know them. If we find out our friends have a trainer, we connect with them; we're always on the prowl.

This means that we've never had to stress about hiring someone; we were able to just look at our network ask someone. If they can't do it, we ask the next person on the list.

'I've tried bringing trainers in before, but my clients don't like them. How do I make it work?'

The simplest way to explain that is they won't like them as much as you – they signed up for you! It's your job to train that trainer up to earn your clients. If you can train that trainer up so your clients do like them almost as much as you, you can hire double as many people. It's on you, not on that trainer.

'Where do you find the money to hire a second person?'

You may not have the money now, but what's going to happen is you're going to get stuck with too many clients and no one to train them. You can say you don't have enough clients to justify bringing someone on board – okay, but do you want to grow? If you always want to stay small, that's fine, just do it yourself. But if you want to get beyond the 15-20 people coming to your session, eventually you're going to need someone you know and trust to help. It's just the cost of doing business, it's an investment.

Action Task

1. Hire a trainer!
2. Look for another trainer!

Bootcamp A s Bootcamp B

Instructor A is a one-person band. They have 20 clients registered and get 10-15 people per session. They can never seem to get more than 25 clients registered. They can't take a holiday, sick day, personal day, or a day off because they are chained to their job. They don't have the money to pay another trainer, and they don't have another trainer they could ask, anyway. They asked another trainer once, but their clients didn't like that trainer.

Instructor B has two trainers working for them as contractors. Instructor B has 40 clients registered and gets 20-25 people coming per session. Having a second trainer at each session helps keep the group under control and adds variety to the session. Instructor B is loving life because they can take a session off if needs be and they can rely on the other trainer for ideas.

More information

This is the sort of content we cover in our Bootcamp CEC courses – to check them out, simply go to our website (www.fitnesseducationonline.com.au). Also make sure you join our community Facebook Group (www.facebook.com/groups/fitnesseducationonline) where we have over 8000 trainers from all over the world discussing these topics.

Seven Figures and Beyond

So far, we've spoken about how to become a six-figure trainer, how to start making $2000 a week, every week from your bootcamp.

That's cool, but if you want to go to the next step it comes down to two things: personal development, and professional development.

If you don't do those two things there, not only will you not move forwards, you're going to go *backwards*. Even if you say, 'I'm happy where I'm at with six figures, I'm not going to keep growing as a person or trainer because I'm happy just to stay where I am.' That won't happen, and you will go backwards.

Professional development refers to things that are going to directly help grow your business, such as a PT doing a TRX course or a kettlebell course. If you're running your own business, you might go and do a sales and marketing course, or you might get a business mentor.

Personal development is a little bit different; these things will help you grow your business, but more indirectly. These are things like how to be more confident, how to believe in yourself, how to be a better listener, how to live a more fulfilled life, how to be happier, etc. Those things are not going to help with your business directly – you're not going to do a course on how to be happier, and then you're a millionaire. It works indirectly, and I've actually found personal development to be more important than professional development, in terms of finance.

What I mean by that is you can do all the fitness courses in the world, but if you don't believe in yourself, if you're not having fun doing what you're doing, if what you're doing doesn't align with your goals and your mission in life, you're only going to get so far. That's why it's important to work on the both of them. There's heaps of different ways you can do it:

Reading

I'm a huge reader, so I read at least an hour every day, usually something to do with either personal development or professional development.

Audio

I love to listen to both podcasts and audiobooks. If I'm driving anywhere, I'm listening to personal/professional development book or podcast.

Courses and conferences

At the time of writing this book, I have attended the National Fitness Conventions in Australia (FILEX), New Zealand (FITEX), and USA (IDEA) for the past three years. This year I attended Social Media Marketing World (in San Diego). At a minimum you should attend your National Convention. It's not even about getting ahead – if you don't go to that, you'll be behind. If you do want to get ahead – go to something outside of your country! The ones in your country will be filled with your competition. If you go outside of your country, you're getting ahead of your competition.

Masterminds

I'm always in both 'paid' and 'free' masterminds. In my paid masterminds, I pay a membership fee to be part of a group and be surrounded by other successful entrepreneurs. In my free masterminds, I meet up every week (set time and location) with my entrepreneur friends and we discuss business.

I look at professional and personal development as an investment, and this is what's helped me get ahead where I think a lot of people have failed. They look at professional and personal development as an expense, 'I've got to spend this much on a course, this much on a convention,' but I love spending money on that sort of stuff. It's no different to investing in shares, or property, or that sort of thing – if you're going to put a $1000 on shares, ideally you want this to make more than $1000 back. Same thing with property – in 30 years' time, you want your property to have increased in value.

You might be wondering how much you should invest, and it all comes down to the level you're at. My opinion is that you should invest something that's a bit of a sacrifice and it hurts, because if you don't, you might not do the work. For example, say you're already making $100,000 a year and you do a $100 course. If that course is rubbish, you're just not going to put in the effort. But say that course costs $10,000 you're going to pay attention, because you don't want to waste that amount of money.

Our Bootcamp Specialist course costs $2000. I can invest in a $20,000 course (and I have before, a $20,000 mastermind) because if all they could do is teach me how to sell one of those a month for the year, I've made my money back *plus* a return on my investment.

If someone's still running bootcamp at the park and charging $5 a head, they're not going to get the same benefit out of that $20,000 mastermind because they're just not structured for it. That person is better off starting with someone who's going to charge them a couple of hundred bucks and teach them some basics on how to get them started.

What's important is that you're climbing up that ladder. That's what I've found with myself. When I started in the industry, I was just doing the basics.

I would get my 20 CECs every two years, and every six months I'd probably spend a couple of hundred bucks on a course, doing maybe 2-3 courses a year. I'd go to FILEX every couple of years, just doing the bare minimum so that my income stayed the same. As soon as I started investing in myself, that's when I saw the jump.

The first business coach I hired cost $1000, $100 a week for 10 weeks. I didn't really like it, I didn't think I was getting that much out of it, but I still remember he showed me one specific strategy that enabled me to get a client registered for 12 months, which covered the cost of the business coaching. So, not only did I basically get free coaching (in a way), I also learned something. I still use some of those strategies from that business coach today.

From there I started to invest a little bit more; I'd do $1000 here, business coaching there, but I was stuck at that level. As soon as I jumped in and started investing in the next level it went up, but then it plateaued again. Then I made the next jump; I invested in a coach for $5000, which was huge at the time. After that, I invested in a $20,000 course, when I was doing a lot better.

Keep going up that ladder, and keep learning. It puts you ahead of the competition, because there's going to be people who are never going to pay that amount. I'm always going to be one-up on those people because I've invested in myself.

FAQ

'I just don't have that kind of money. What can I do?'

If you want to be successful, you need to do one of two things: you need to invest your money, or you need to invest your time. If you don't have the money, you've got to spend your time (unless you can cut some costs and live cheaply for the next couple of weeks or months to save up some cash, or pick up extra work).

Until then, start with the free stuff. Read books, like the ones I've been recommending at the end of each chapter. Contact us for more suggestions, or for links to the podcasts and audiobooks we listen to.

'How do we know if the investment, or the coach, is worth it?'

Like with any investment, there's no guarantee. The only way is to give it a crack, and try to minimise the risk. Check out reviews, research the coach, have a chat to them, and see if it aligns with what you want to do.

It comes down to the risk-reward ratio. If you're going to do something, there's always an element of risk involved. That's why you'll be successful. If there's no risk involved, everybody would do it, and then it's not going to be special. But if you're the one who can take that risk, you've knocked out half your competition already.

'How do you find the time? My books are full!'

If your books are full and you're happy, that's great. Keep doing what you're doing. But if you want to grow, you're going to have to make a sacrifice – cut something out so that you can make room to grow.

Action Task

1. Hire a mentor/coach to help take you to the next level of your life.

Afterword

Congratulations on finishing this book! You're in the top level of achievers, so we want to give you a reward for reading to the end. To claim your free gift, just email Jono at jonathon@fitnesseducationonline.com.au.

If you've learned something from this book, that's great, but we've got a bit of a different goal for you. What's important is that you implement what you learn. A lot of people say knowledge is power, but we completely disagree. Knowledge is only *potential* power. You need to action that knowledge to make it power. If there's one thing we recommend more than anything else, take action.

If you're not sure where to start, there's a couple of different ways to do it. If you've been highlighting and taking notes on the way, that's great, implement those notes. If you haven't, just read it again in more detail, highlight what you need to, write down notes. Work your way through the whole book.

Keep this book with you, so that whenever you're stuck on bootcamp problems, you'll have the answers right there with you. If you need anything more, just reach out to us.

About Jono

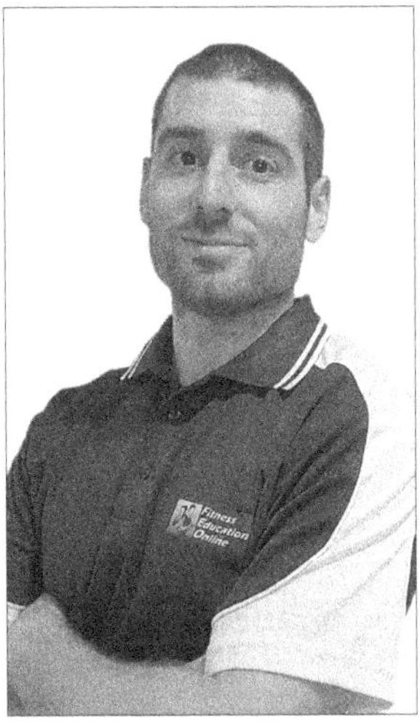

Jono is a personal trainer and Exercise Physiologist from Sydney, Australia. Upon graduating in 2008, Jono started working in different gyms across Sydney.

In 2012, Jono transitioned from personal training in gyms to running outdoor bootcamps, which he soon discovered was his passion.

Jono dedicated the next six years of his life to becoming the best bootcamp instructor in the world by completing courses, going to conferences and conventions, hiring coaches, and immersing himself in bootcamps online and in real life. He was soon able to generate a full income running one bootcamp session a day, and absolutely loved it!

While Jono was running his bootcamp, he would speak to other trainers who weren't able to make a full time income in the fitness industry, and were forced to leave doing what they loved and go back to a full-time job which they hated. It broke his heart that other people weren't able to do the same as he had done. He connected with his good childhood friend, Travis Mattern, and they created Fitness Education Online.

Fitness Education Online has connected more than 5000 trainers across Australia, New Zealand, UK, and USA with their bootcamp Courses. They have spoken at the biggest fitness conventions across Australia and New Zealand (FILEX and FITEX), and hosted the #1 podcast for personal trainers wanting to grow their bootcamp, titled *The Bootcamp Blueprint*. They are the foremost experts in helping personal trainers grow their bootcamp.

Contact them via the links below:

www.fitnesseducationonline.com.au

jonathon@fitnesseducationonline.com.au

Facebook: www.facebook.com/jono.petrohilos

Instagram: @jono_petrohilos

About Travis

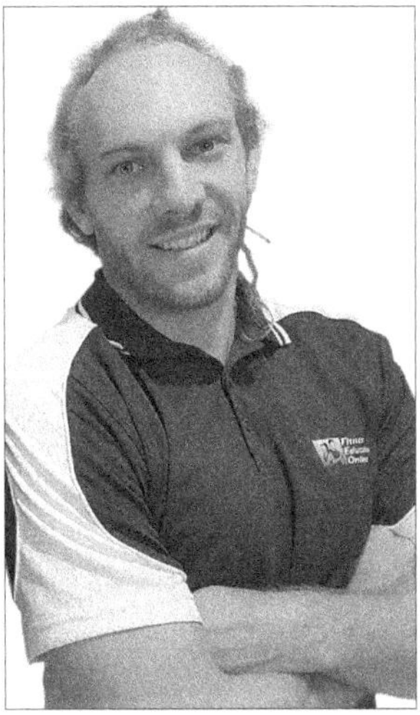

I have always been active, and love being involved in competition, something I have missed as I've gotten a little older.

I am the third of four brothers, so we were always wrestling and rumbling around the house. One year we were given boxing gloves and just told by our mum to 'Go for it, just don't hit each other in the head'. Obviously, a few stray shots got through every now and again!

I did gymnastics for about 15 years, and coached for about five years, even in the USA. I have also competed in other sports such as tennis, swimming, cricket, rugby league, rugby union, AFL, soccer, touch football, and more recently Brazilian Jiu Jitsu.

I love teaching and coaching, and over the last 15 years I have worked in some way as a coach or mentor. I completed a Bachelor of Education and commenced work in primary school, and ran various school sports programs and coached a number of different sporting teams. Meanwhile I completed my Certificate III and IV in Fitness, working in both a commercial gym setting and outdoor bootcamp setting. I have since gone on to specialise in Functional Training, and have written various courses on kettlebells, suspension training, medicine balls, powerbags, resistance bands, and bootcamps. I have been lucky enough to be able to travel the world to learn from industry leaders in the various fields.

For anyone reading this, thank you! I hope you are able to use the content provided to follow your own path and create something special yourselves. Being in the fitness industry is often very difficult, and the lifespan of a trainer is usually very short. We burn ourselves out trying to help everybody; getting up early, finishing late, not taking holidays, and generally putting everybody before ourselves. I hope the methods provided in this book allow you to solve some of these issues and create a bootcamp that is not only sustainable for your health, but also profitable.

Thanks again,

Travis Mattern

travis@fitnesseducationonline.com.au

www.fitnesseducationonline.com.au

IG: @travis_the_kettlebell_guy

Acknowledgments

We'd like to specifically thank our mentors, who have helped us along our journey:

- Brenda Romaniello
- April Barcenal
- Ashy Evans
- Steve Evans
- Levi Walz
- AJ Mihrzad
- Matt Kazam
- Natasa Denman

We recommended reading ...

- *Advanced Selling Strategies* by Brian Tracey
- *Awaken the Giant Within* by Anthony Robbins
- *Be Obsessed or Be Average* by Grant Cardone
- *Building a Story Brand* by Donald Miller
- *Common Denominator of Success* by Albert E Gray
- *Dotcom Secrets* by Russel Brunson
- *How to Win Friends and Influence People* by Dale Carnegie
- *Influence* by Robert Cialdini
- *Launch* by Jeff Walker
- *Membership Economy* by Robbie Kellman Baxter
- *Million Dollar Habits* by Brian Tracey
- *Negotiation* by Brian Tracey
- *No BS Direct Marketing* by Dan Kennedy
- *Raving Fans* by Ken Blanchard

- *Rich Dad Poor Dad* by Robert Kiyosaki
- *Rich Habits Poor Habits* by Tom Corley and Michael Yardley
- *Secrets of Closing the Sale* by Zig Ziglar
- *See You at the Top* by Zig Ziglar
- *Sell or Be Sold* by Grant Cardone
- *Stop Acting Rich* by Thomas Stanley
- *The 10X Rule* by Grant Cardone
- *The 4 Hour Work Week* by Timothy Ferris
- *The Greatest Salesmen in the World* by OG Mandino
- *The Millionaire Mind* by Thomas J Stanley
- *The Psychology of Selling* by Brian Tracey
- *The Richest Man in Babylon* by George Clason
- *The Secret* by Rhona Byrne
- *The Success Principles* by Jack Canfield
- *Think and Grow Rich* by Napolean Hill
- *You Don't Have to Be Born Brilliant* by John McGrath
- *You Were Born Rich* by Bob Proctor

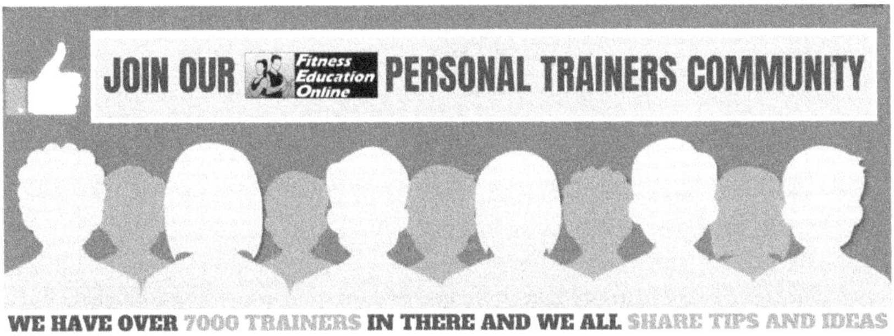

Your Tribe Affects Your Vibe!

Fitness Education Online have a community Facebook Group with more than 8000 members. It is a very supportive community, and we all share tips and ideas! We would love for you to be a part of our community.

To join simply visit www.facebook.com/groups/fitnesseducationonline, or search Fitness Education Online Community in the Facebook search bar (note: make sure to 'join the group' as opposed to liking the page).

BONUS: Every person who joins our community Facebook Group also receives a FREE copy of our course *Fitness Games for Bootcamp*.

Jono and Travis, the co-directors at Fitness Education Online are highly sought after, international professional speakers. They have presented at the biggest fitness conventions in Australia and New Zealand (FILEX and FITEX).

They are both university-educated in Exercise Physiology and Education, respectively, and have more than 20 years' experience in the fitness industry.

Through their online courses, they have helped more than 5000 trainers take their fitness business to the next level.

These courses are registered in Australia (Fitness Australia, Physical Activity Australia, and FITREC), New Zealand (REPS), and United States of America (ACE and NASM).

Topic 1: Bootcamp Blueprint: How Personal Trainers Can Make 6 Figures a Year Working 60mins a Day!

» Why bootcamp is your best option.
» How to create bootcamps that sell.
» How to never lose a client again.

Topic 2: Bootcamp Workout Ideas

» How to create unlimited workout ideas using limited equipment.
» Equipment myths: you don't need to spend thousands of dollars on equipment.
» The one-percenters that make all the difference.

Topic 3: Social Media Essentials for Trainers

» How to get as many clients as you want
» It's not who you know, it's who knows you
» Make money while you sleep

Courses registered with:

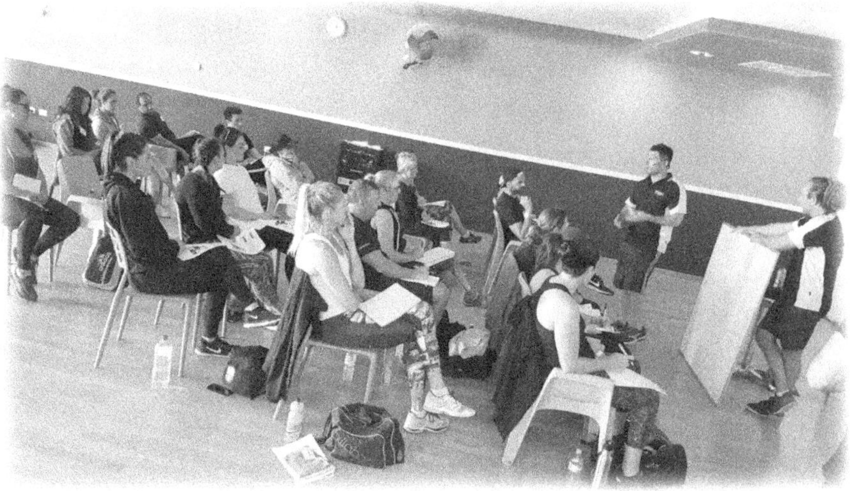

Contact *Jono:*

www.fitnesseducationonline.com.au

jonathon@fitnesseducationonline.com.au

Facebook: www.facebook.com/jono.petrohilos

Instagram: @jono_petrohilos

Contact Travis:

travis@fitnesseducationonline.com.au

www.fitnesseducationonline.com.au

Instagram: @travis_the_kettlebell_guy

Fitness Education Online

Does this sound like you? Are you still

- wanting to grow that bootcamp, but not sure where to start?
- not sure how to attract your ideal clients?
- struggling to get exposure and be an authority in your area?
- tired of being the best kept secret in your area?
- sick of sharing your gift, giving every client 110%, and working your butt off without receiving sufficient income?
- confused on how to package and position so you can charge what your worth?
- feeling stagnant with regard to growing your business?
- lacking guidance from an experienced mentor?

Becoming the go-to bootcamp trainer in your area changes everything. If more people know about you, you'll be able to change more lives and increase your income dramatically.

At Fitness Education Online we have a large array of internationally recognised courses and programs that are all specifically designed to helping personal trainers grow their bootcamp.

Find more info at:

www.fitnesseducationonline.com.au

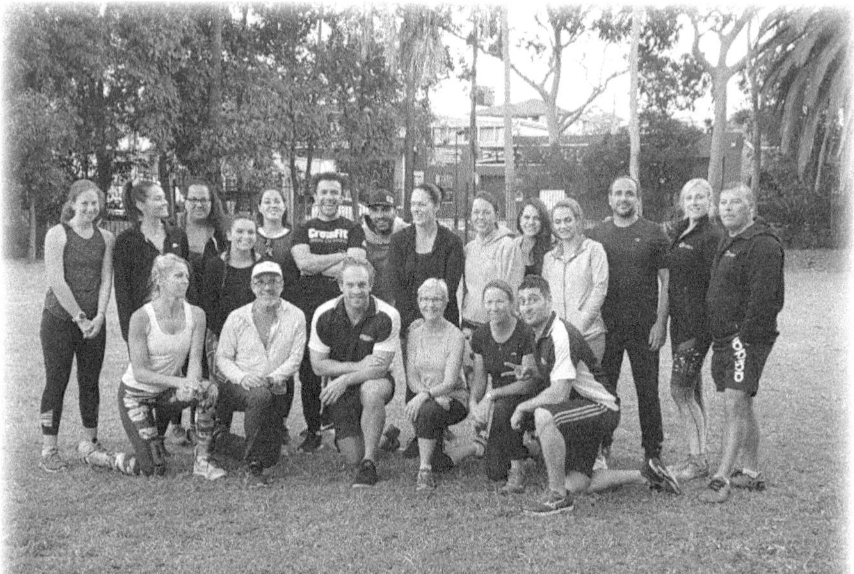

CPSIA information can be obtained
at www.ICGtesting.com
Printed in the USA
BVHW030517011121
620436BV00008B/284

9 781925 830347